The Genesis Factor

The Genesis Factor
Diet and Fitness for a New Beginning

Dr. Ben Lerner

New York Times, Wall Street Journal, USA Today,
and Christian Booksellers Association best-selling author of
the groundbreaking Christian wellness book, *Body By God*

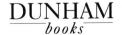

Trade Paperback ISBN: 978-0-9851359-7-3
Ebook ISBN: 978-0-9855328-3-3

Printed in the United States of America

Contents

Foreword

Dr. Ben Lerner has redefined the way that we look at health, wellness, and by extension one's own mentality.

We are products of our environment, and what we put into our bodies directly affects the way that we feel and the way that we act. 1 Corinthians 6:19 tells us, "Do you not know that your bodies are temples of the Holy Spirit, who is in you, whom you have received from God?" (NIV) Life is the most precious gift we have, and to honor God and be responsible caretakers of that life is our greatest duty.

There is a renewed focus on health and wellness breaking through the body of Christ, and Dr. Ben Lerner and Maximized Living are on the forefront of that movement. To obey God requires a full commitment of mind, body, and soul.

I spoke at the Maximized Living seminar in Denver, Colorado in September 2013. Dr. Lerner and I agreed on opening a Maximized Living Health Center through the Maximized Living Foundation at The Dream Center. We did exactly what we committed to do, and the impact this has had on our residents, staff, volunteers, and the tens of thousands of people in the community that we serve has gone beyond my wildest imagination.

I am amazed at the testimonials of the people who have visited the Maximized clinic. Literally, every time I walk through The Dream Center, someone comes up to tell me how the work done at the clinic has changed or touched their life in some profound and positive way.

One young lady tried over and over to turn her life around, even dropping out of the program several times. Now she says, "This time I can do it! The care and education I get at the clinic will give me the strength and ability to beat my addictions."

Another individual told me the reason this has changed his life is that they teach and explain the "Why" of taking care of your body in a way that has allowed him to finally make the lifestyle changes he needs to live the abundant life Christ came to give him.

These are just two of the many, many testimonials that I have heard due to this great service Dr. Lerner and the Maximized Living Foundation are providing.

The generosity of the Maximized Living Foundation has been incredible. They use brand new, state-of-the-art equipment including an x-ray machine with the latest technology. The quality and quantity of care and education provided is the same at The Dream Center as in all of their hundreds of for-profit clinics around the world.

When I give tours of The Dream Center, I can't wait to take everyone to the Health Center to show off the quality of the doctors, staff, and the equipment there and to tell them the difference this organization is making in The Dream Center.

In addition, The Maximized Living Foundation has now opened a salad bar for all the residents of The Dream Center along with the homeless that come to the Food Chapel for a warm meal.

The Foundation not only teaches our residents about the right nutrition but also supplies fresh fruits and vegetables every day. For some of these people, it's the first consistent nutrients they've ever received in their entire lives.

Together with Dr. Lerner and The Dream Center, we will continue to allow people to "Dream again."

This work has changed my life, is changing millions of lives, and will change your life as well.

Take the Genesis Challenge, and change your life for God as well.

—Pastor Matthew Barnett
Senior Pastor, Angelus Temple
and Co-founder of The Dream Center

In The Beginning . . .

Wholeness Ministry—How This "Whole" Journey Began

Before I explain just exactly what the "Genesis Factor" is and how it's going to renew your whole body to its highest level, I need to set the stage for how wellness connects with a life in Christ and briefly inspire you to jump onboard.

So, here's how it started...

When my youngest brother was "busy being born," my parents left me with our very Catholic next-door neighbors. As a result, I ended up going to church for my very first time... ever.

The church was huge, and our Italian-Catholic neighborhood seemed to literally be built as a secondary thought around this massive religious institution. Now, as a 9-year-old boy, walking through those gigantic wooden doors for the very first time, I was mesmerized by the herculean-sized statue of Jesus Christ.

Instantly, I was awe-struck by one sole feature of this statue...

Jesus was *ripped*!

He didn't just have a 6-pack—He had a 14-pack!!

I immediately went home and informed my very non-Christian parents, "I want to be like Jesus!" You can imagine how that went over.

Most people take religion and put it in one box, and then they place health and fitness in an entirely different one. Yet, we truly aren't fragmented beings like that.

We are one—body, mind, and spirit. And as a result, each area impacts the others. It's all interconnected. In the church, health isn't being ripped like Jesus. Instead, it's being good stewards with our bodies for many reasons. We are to honor the gift of health, find the energy to serve God's purposes, and live for Christ, our family, and the people that are counting on us. It's not just about abs.

As we know, Christ's ministry is about God's deep love and compassion for people. God profoundly considers all the details of your life in a way that exceeds your comprehension – including your health and vitality.

Your wellbeing is of great importance to Him! He explains in the Scriptures, *"Beloved, I wish above all things that thou mayest prosper and be in health, even as thy soul prospereth."* (3 John 1:2)

We know that Jesus is the primary purpose of the Bible and the Gospel, and… "The main thing is to keep the main thing the main thing."

And… the "main thing" is Jesus!

But, there's also the compassion part of Christ's ministry or what is known as the "Second Hand of the Gospel." This encompasses God caring for the wellbeing of His children, including the food they eat, and yes, their physical and mental health. In fact, did you know that in Jesus' narration of His ministry in Matthew, 83% of it has to do with keeping us alive and well? That's right!

When John the Baptist was imprisoned and aware of his impending death, he pleaded with his disciples to quickly go make sure that Jesus was "The One."

When asked, Jesus answered, *"Go, and show John those things which you hear and see: The blind receive their sight, and the lame walk, the lepers are cleansed, the deaf hear, the dead are raised up, and the poor have the gospel preached to them."* (Matthew 11:4-5)

Five out of the six things He used to describe His work touched on your health and aliveness!

As our Father, God really cares—and He knows you'll have a pretty tough time here on Earth serving Him or your family and enjoying life if you're sick or dead. As the pirates say, "Dead men tell no tales." Clearly, the wellbeing of people was a major part of Christ's ministry – and should still be a central theme today, so His people can live out a better testimony.

Thankfully, many pastors, ministry leaders, and CEOs around the world are dedicated to the same amazing cause that we are. Our doctors passionately lead hundreds of health and wholeness ministries and corporate wellness programs reaching hundreds of thousands of people each year. Projects I've created such as Rebuild the Temple and Winning My Race have been followed by many key Christian movements like Elevation Church in Charlotte, North Carolina and The Dream Center in Los Angeles, California.

I've written over a dozen other books either personally or with the expert help of many other talented Maximized Living doctors. For years, people have asked me to "Just tell them what to eat and how to get in shape. Nothing else." And that is exactly what I've done here!

However, if you want additional information on nutrition and exercise or want to know the "why" behind the details and plans contained here, go to www.maximizedliving.com or contact one of our Maximized Living doctor's offices around the globe.

Chapter 1
Our Natural *"Body by God"*

Nothing is impossible. The word itself says I'm possible.
—Audrey Hepburn

For nothing is impossible with God. —Luke 1:37

Think about it. 7-11, Arby's, Hot-Pockets, couches, computers, plasma TV, the Internet, Starbucks, and home delivery are certainly a far cry from walking with God in the cool of the day, naming animals, and plucking grapes in your backyard like Adam and Eve did. So, the questions that spring to the forefront of our minds now are:

- "How did they survive without Starbucks?"
- "How did they know anything without Googling it?"
- "How did they find their way around the garden without their iPhone maps app?"

It almost seems out of order, doesn't it? With God being all-knowing like He is and because He loves us so much, you'd think that on the 6th day, He would've...

- Created the iPhone, the Internet, Pizza Hut, Wal-Mart, Dunkin' Donuts, tanning beds, Lazy-Boy, and IKEA;
- Taken the 7th day off;
- and then on the 8th day, created man.

From today's standards, we certainly seem to have been born about two thousand years too early, right?

Or, perhaps, Fried Oreos, Sweet Tarts, Lipitor, Diet Coke, triple mocha lattes, and Captain Crunch weren't part of the plan (I hope I'm not making anyone hungry!).

The good news is, no matter where you are with your health today, you can be made new—or at least "new-er" by tapping into the Genesis Factor.

In this program, we're going to reveal to you the best, *easiest*, and *fastest* possible ways to maximize fitness, optimize leanness, and eat right for your hormones—all as an essential plan to upgrade and/or restore wellness.

Chapter 2
Made New
What was health to Jesus?

Life is like a ten-speed bike. Most of us have gears we never use. —Charles Schultz

Brothers and sisters, God has shown you his mercy. So I am asking you to offer up your bodies to him while you are still alive. Your bodies are a holy sacrifice that is pleasing to God. When you offer your bodies to God, you are worshiping him.
—Romans 12:1

The Genesis Factor at Work
In your quest to get and stay well, your first question should be, "What does 'well' look like to Jesus?"

According to the Gospel of John, there was a pool by a Sheep Gate called Bethesda. The disabled, the blind, the lame, the paralyzed, and the sick would come lie by it, and the legend was that an angel would come stir the waters. Then, the first one in the pool would be healed.

In John 5, Jesus sees a man who has been an invalid for 38 years lying by this pool, and He asks the man, "Do you wish to get well?"

For getting well, Jesus uses the Greek words, *Genesthai Hoog-yace.*

Genestathai: you'll recognize this word from the Bible and the name of this book. It comes from the term "Genesis" which means created, generation, or beginning.

Hoogyace: this means sound or whole.

So, when Jesus says "get well," He's literally saying:

- Are you committed to being re-generated?
- Do you wish to be restored whole?
- Would you like a new beginning?
- Are you ready to be made new?

Unlike our quick fixers today, Jesus doesn't do pain relief, medication distribution, surgery, or symptom treatment. He's looking for you to be re-created whole and live the life you were re-born to live.

Your Genesis Factor means:
- You can be made new!
- You can be restored!
- You can be made whole and get your form back.
- Jesus is looking for you to do it, and He's ready to help!

This Genesis Factor doesn't just make biblical sense. It makes scientific sense as well. Every day, millions of cells are dying and being replaced by millions of new ones. But did you know that if put in the wrong state, living the wrong lifestyle—dying, sick cells are replaced by more dying, sick cells?

The good news is that if you've been building disease and fat, through the principle of the Genesis Factor, you can now build health and burn fat. It's God's physiological grace and metabolic mercy.

God's Universal Laws

The context for the Genesis Factor is the setting of the book of Genesis itself. It's based upon the realization that we were originally created by God and placed in a beautiful, plentiful, and natural setting to thrive as His children. So, because our foundation is of natural substance, when we put artificial substances in our body, the results are... you've got it... unnatural!

There are natural laws of the Universe that God Himself has put in place.

For example, there are chemical laws. If you combine sodium (Na) and chloride (Cl), you get salt. If you combine $2H + 1O$, you get H^2O (or water). However, if you combine 2 H's and 2 O's, it creates hydrogen peroxide—which is not nearly as refreshing. A slight change can make a huge difference!

There are also physical laws. If you jump off of a ten-story building and pray for God to catch you... while God can do anything... you'll likely experience His laws of physics and how they apply when human matter moving at terminal velocity of 122 mph meets an immovable force—i.e. the ground. The results are unpleasant.

In fact, you'd most likely get to meet God quickly after, and you could ask Him, "Father, why didn't you catch me?"

To which, He'll likely reply, "I gave you a brain and an eighth-grade physics teacher, dummy, so you'd know not to jump!"

It's exactly the same concept when you consistently eat food He didn't mean for you to eat. You're out of shape, your spine is degenerating, and you're vitamin and mineral deficient—you're breaking God's physical laws.

Praying for God's healing while ignoring various parts of your lifestyle is the same as praying for God to catch you when you jump off of the building.

While He can—and, in some cases, does—do some amazing things to help His children who get sidetracked in a big way, the results of a destructive lifestyle are generally undesirable, to say the least.

As I called my first book, you really do have a *Body by God*. So, it has become crystal clear over time that the further you stray from the lifestyle you were created to live, the sicker, fatter, and more painful, sleepless, and depressed you become. This is one of the main reasons why you're told to "*Honor God with your body.*" (1 Corinthians 6:19-20)

Thankfully, wherever you are at today, you can be restored, and take your body and your health to whatever level necessary to fulfill your destiny.

The diet and fitness plans I'll show you here are designed to restore good hormones, reduce disease-causing inflammation, start burning fat, and help you to reverse or slow the effects of aging. A plan, through the grace God extended you in your body, to quite literally provide you with a new beginning.

God's Wellness Plan

What does God's wellness plan entail? Have you ever heard of Sir Robert Augustus Chesebrough? He was the inventor of Vaseline and lived to 96 years old. He believed his secret for longevity was eating a tablespoon of Vaseline a day. This is not going to release your Genesis Factor.

Ever eaten processed foods? Who hasn't, right? I once read the ingredients on a bag of blueberry bagels, and to my surprise, there were no actual blueberries on the label. All it said was, "Blue and purple colored chips." Nothing with blue and purple coloring are on the Genesis Foods List.

So... what does incorporate the right principles? A better example was Jack LaLanne, an early Christian pioneer for health. In his 90s, he was still pulling tugboats—with his teeth. He understood wholeness when he said, "If God didn't make it, I won't eat it." Now that's a principle in alignment with the power of the Genesis Factor available within you! If you place artificial substances inside your "body by God" or do things to disturb its ability to function properly, then you are stimulating hundreds of thousands of negative counter-reactions.

However, the good news is: God is our Father of amazing grace.

And if you provide your temple (body) with the care and nourishment that aligns with His intentions, you can heal, sustain, and live the kind of life you desire. Thus, your new beginning....

Chapter 3
God's Myth Busters Revealed
Kiss Melba goodbye!

Our greatest glory is not in never failing, but in rising up every time we fall. —Ralph Waldo Emerson

Don't you know that your bodies are temples of the Holy Spirit? The Spirit is in you. You have received him from God. You do not belong to yourselves. Christ has paid the price for you. So use your bodies in a way that honors God." —1 Corinthians 6:19-20

Living the Genesis Factor Every Day

My wife and I are living examples of the Genesis Factor at work. Health and fitness are foundational in our home. I'm always trying to set a new fitness record, and my wife is always working to get back to her original weight—7lbs and 4oz.

My wife qualified for the 70.3 (half ironman) World Championships at age 48, and at 47, I beat my marathon time from when I was 29 years old by 90 minutes. We can't wait to see what 50 holds for us!

We have thousands of stories from people of all ages—professionals, Olympic athletes, and entire families who are succeeding in our programs all around the world.

On the other hand, growing up, my family really struggled with their health, weight, and exercise (or lack thereof). My parents, aunts, and uncles are all from New York, home of the majority of bad carbs—New York Cheesecake, New York Pizza, New York Bakery, and New York Bagels, etc.

Eating well was a real challenge back in my parents' day. Good nutrition meant going on a "diet" and only eating celery, carrot sticks, cottage cheese, and the driest substance on earth—Melba toast. Although I haven't eaten Melba toast since 1981, I can still taste it. I'm not sure who Melba was, but she makes some pretty nasty toast.

Unfortunately, my family's problem wasn't just diet-based—exercise was a problem as well. In New York City, if you were running, it wasn't exercise—it was because someone was chasing you. My parents hated exercise. In our house, we could say swear words, but we weren't allowed to say "exercise."

Ultimately, it seemed almost impossible for anyone in our family to be lean and healthy. My father died at 52, and my mother became permanently disabled by a stroke at 49. So, I've made health and wellness my ministry and am giving you the secrets I've discovered through my lifelong journey into health.

One reason people fail is all the myths they believe that shackle them versus the truths that will set them free. My life experiences have shown me, we've got to start by setting the record straight.

Public Myths Vs. Genesis Truths

There are many 'nutritional myths' floating around out there, and part of the Genesis Factor is identifying the truths that will set you free.

MYTH #1: Eat like an elephant, look like an elephant.

TRUTH: If you are eating the foods God intended you to, you won't look like an elephant. Like most people, I need a diet in which I can eat all I want and still look and feel desirable. To *eat like an elephant, but look like a ripped deer*. In our Advance Plan, you can eat all you want! You only need to reduce quantities based on how far you deviate from the program.

MYTH #2: If you crave, you cave.

TRUTH: Taking short vacations from proper eating is part of the plan. So, if you cheat or get off track, it's not "Game Over" for you.

MYTH #3: "Low-," "Reduced-," "-free," and "No-" foods are health and diet food. And foods that are good for you are expensive.

TRUTH: Synthetic, refined, or chemically altered foods that say "Low-fat," "Reduced-cholesterol," "Lactose-free," "Sugar-free," etc., will never grant long-term health or thinness and are expensive. Simply put, anything man creates for you to eat cannot be considered "health and diet food."

Food by God is the only health and diet food there is! And overall, it costs a lot less. So, wave good-bye to worldly nutritional myths and frustration…and say hello to your new Genesis Factor lifestyle!

"The Genesis Factor" Eating Made Timely, Easy, and Affordable

Taste and Price

Typically, when you think of the foods you are allowed to shovel into your mouth, you think, *Yucky…and pricey!* I was exactly the same way. That is why, for even the most inexperienced of healthy eaters, the meals and snacks we recommend taste great. Buying natural foods in bulk is extremely cheap when compared to eating out or purchasing prepackaged foods.

Health food stores and lots of grocery stores carry organic foods. Organic items—particularly meats and dairy—will help keep your diet largely free of chemicals. While, organic food can be expensive, it will save you thousands of dollars on medical care.

Ease

Since these are prepared meals, always cook enough to eat for more than one meal. That way when you're "on-the-go," you can pack your healthy meals to prevent being stranded without healthy options. But who has the time for all this? You do! To make it super easy, we've got this all laid out in food guides for breakfast/lunch/dinner/snacks/desserts, meal plans, shopping lists, and recipes.

It's All About Hormones

Regeneration means you must master the *hormone factor.* Hormones aren't simply a matter of age, luck, or genetics. They're a result of lifestyle. In a nutshell, exercise, diet, and hormone patterns are the reason "couch potatoes" eventually end up looking like . . . the couch. With hormones, the sooner you act the better. Your sedentary, simple carb life from birth to 10 years of age will come back and haunt you at 30. A teenage, fast food, technology-oriented lifestyle will make you fat at 40.

Starting at 30, 40, 50 years of age or later? Don't worry, it's not too late—we've got food and exercise secrets to help or even reverse any hormone problems you've created. It's all part of the plan, so, let's get started!

Chapter 4

Food by God Or Food by Man?
If God didn't make it, don't eat it!

It's not that I'm so smart, it's just that I stay with problems longer. —Albert Einstein

Let us not become weary in doing good, for at the proper time we will reap a harvest if we do not give up. —Galatians 6:9

Food... as God Intended It

When God developed the body, He specifically created certain foods for its nourishment. These are the foods that grow and exist in nature—"Food by God." Within these foods, He has supplied everything that is necessary, in just the right amounts, and in the perfect balance needed, for proper digestion, distribution, and elimination of nutrients.

The farther away any product is from its natural state, the way God made it, the more potentially harmful it is. When you take in "Food by God" in its natural state, the digestive system far more readily breaks it down, dispenses the nutrients to body cells, and quickly eliminates leftover toxins and by-products.

Man-Made Food

"Food by Man" is food that is created or altered by man and that God did not design for the express purpose of being consumed or processed by your body on a regular basis. Yes, French fries, although once a potato, do sadly fall into this category.

As we can see in today's society, "Food by Man" has a constant negative effect on the body. So even if someone says, "Where's the proof that some artificial sweetener or boxed up, refined *Lunchable* isn't healthy?" Tell them the proof is in their artificially flavored, chemically colored, thickening agent filled, sugar-free, diet-pudding.

When a Natural Thing May not be a "God-Thing"

There's talk in the Bible of eating meat, milk, bread, and honey. However, their meat source was eating grass on a farm, the milk on their tables was fresh from under the cow, the wheat in their bread wasn't a mutated clone, and they didn't mainline sugar like we do today.

Raise an animal differently than God intended, manipulate a once natural crop, or overdo carbohydrates, and there are real dangers that God did not intend to come across your path. The consequences are inflammation, diabetes, weight gain, rapid aging, and subsequent degenerative disease.

As the old commercial for margarine used to say, "It's not nice to fool Mother Nature." Of course, it turns out margarine is really fake butter that is really bad for you.

The Hormone Effect—How "Fat" Happens

In reality, gaining weight is a marker of too much carb energy and the growing inability of your body's hormones to manage all the sugar and the excess fat the sugar creates. Since the intake of more sugar than your body can manage causes obesity and obesity-related diseases, like diabetes, high triglycerides, bad cholesterol, and advanced aging, it makes sense to say, "Carbs Kill." Because I know first-hand that curbing the carbs is no easy task, I will give you plenty of tools to make the necessary improvements.

Your tools will include: the Genesis Foods List, meal plans and recipes, the Carb Counter, and plenty of allowable desserts. Now we're talking, right?

Chapter 5
Baby, We Were Born to Run
Why furniture doesn't exist in nature!

When deeds speak, words are nothing.—African Proverb

But someone will say, "You have faith; I have deeds." Show me your faith without deeds, and I will show you my faith by my deeds.
—James 2:18

You can't just swallow health. In the beginning, God gave us muscles, a heart, and lungs. You might wonder, "Why did He do that?" We are given muscles and various energy systems in order to:

- Walk or jog great distances
- Get up mountains
- Run from danger
- Serve a purpose

Most people have been taught to believe that if you're thinner or lighter it means you're healthier. But, the truth is, if you just starve yourself, follow some weird diet, take pills, or do bariatric surgery, you may lose weight, *but you'll just die lighter.*

In reality, it's only when reaching a more ideal weight is accompanied by your cardiovascular system (heart, lungs, and blood vessels) efficiently handling oxygen and having a good ratio of muscle mass versus fat mass (loosely packed muscle) that you are actually getting healthier.

Plus, like Adam and Eve, you'll look good naked—or at least not too bad in fig leaves.

Heart and lung function along with optimal body composition (a high muscle-to-fat ratio) are critical survival needs that can't be improved through diets, pills, potions, drugs, surgery, or electric stimulation alone. No matter what the infomercial tells you, *to serve God with all your strength,* you'll have to actually move.

Exercise for many is emotional. By that, I mean, they actually hate exercise. Pretty extreme. But by learning about a new program that allows you to get in great shape by implementing only 12 minute routines and signing up for a race, I'm hoping to get you moving and turn this emotion into love rather than hate (or at least "like").

Chapter 6
The Genesis Challenge

It is not because things are difficult that we do not dare; it is because we do not dare that things are difficult. —Seneca

Where there is no revelation, people cast off restraint; but blessed is the one who heeds wisdom's instruction.
                                        —Proverbs 29:18

If you remember from John 5, "get well" to Jesus is a Greek version of Genesis—restored, a new beginning. Jesus says to the sick man, "Do you wish... to be restored?"

Now, think about this. The man had been an invalid for 38 years. So, why would Jesus say, "Do you wish....?" It seems like He's asking a ridiculous question. This man had lived his life lying on a pallet for almost four decades—of course the man would want to get better—right?

However, since Jesus only asks supernaturally great questions, we have to look at what does "Do you wish" mean. The Greek word here for wish is "thélō." This word, in this context, really means purpose or intention. Another level up from *wish*.

So, when we break it down, we find that Jesus was really asking if the man was committed. Ultimately He was saying, "Are you really intending to make wholeness, through Me, your purpose—to take on the Genesis challenge?"

The commitment to this challenge can be intimidating. In fact, the disabled man, even knowing it would save his life, didn't say yes. Instead he responds to Jesus, "Sir, I have no one to help me into the pool when the water is stirred."

Instead of taking on the Genesis challenge, he fired off an excuse, and then quite literally blamed the healthcare system. Yet, full of mercy and grace, Jesus took great delight in healing him. Thankfully, Jesus' commitment to His purpose always exceeds ours and fills in the gaps where needed.

Christ is asking all of us the same question, "*Will you take the Genesis challenge?* Are you committed to being restored whole?"

Don't be like the guy at the pool. My hope is that your answer will be, "Yes—I'll take the Challenge and make wellness part of my purpose!"

My desire for you is renewal, where you will become everything you were re-born to be. I pray that you will have the health, time, and energy to finish the assignment God has given you and fulfill your destiny.

It's my goal that millions take the Genesis Challenge and experience their Genesis Factor—starting right now!

Releasing Your Genesis Factor
The 30 Days to Advanced Eating and Run for Hope Training Plans

Difficult things take time. Impossible things just a little longer.
—Author Unknown

Everything is possible for one who believes. —Mark 9:23

Further down in this chapter, you will see that we've provided 30 days of advanced meal plans along with a shopping guide and all of the recipes you need—and then some. This is a hormone-based diet that allows you to eat desserts every day (and more than once a day). It is designed to help you reach goals like: losing weight, getting lean, detoxifying your body, and radically reducing inflammation and inflammatory disease.

If, after 30 days, you've reached your goals, you can begin to add in Core Plan foods from the Genesis Food List. However, many people enjoy the Advanced Plan so much because they feel and look so good that they stay on the Advanced Plan (with vacation meals) for life. That's what my wife and I did.

The Run for Hope:
Be a Hero by Getting in Shape to Fulfill God's Purposes

No matter where you're starting from, I've created training programs to complete a 5K, 10K, Half-Marathon, and Marathon. There's nothing like signing up for a race to get your "fitness groove" on.

If you really want to get fit for a cause, you can do what The Dream

Center in Los Angeles does. They participate in the LA 5K and Marathon race each year to raise money for the fight against Human Trafficking. People can even do the marathon as a two person relay and just run a half marathon.

We're utilizing the training programs here to help their cause, and hopefully, this will help you do the same in your neck of the woods. Find your own local charity to support, and go from the couch—or your current state of fitness—into one of these running races. You'll not only get in the best shape of your life, but you'll help save lives as well! It's a win-win! (See all of the information on The Dream Center Run for Hope Challenge in Appendix V.)

Take on one or both parts (food and fitness) of the Challenge—either way, you're putting your Genesis Factor to work!

By taking the Challenge and following the meal and/or the training plans, you'll experience first-hand what it feels like to get the Genesis Factor working in your life. Take on both parts of the challenge or do them separately. Either way, you're going to enjoy another level of wholeness and restoration and become better equipped to fulfill your destiny.

Additional Nutrition Guidelines for the different distance races can be found with the training plans.

30-Days to Advanced Eating
Our Core and Advanced Plans

One may go a long way after one is tired. —French Proverb

I can do all things through Christ who strengthens me.
                                                    —Philippians 4:13

The Genesis Challenge is designed to show you exactly how to eat and exercise to change your life over the next few weeks. For more information on nutrition and exercise, explore our resources at maximizedliving.com, or visit one of our Maximized Living doctor's offices around the globe.

The Advanced Plan
Our Advanced Plan is a no grain, no sugar, and low carb plan. It's hormonally sound eating that will help you to detox, re-boot your good hormones, and reduce pain and disease-causing inflammation. Advanced eating effectively reverses the effect of the S.A.D. (Standard American Diet).

The 30 Days to Advanced Eating Meal Plans are based on the Advanced Plan. This plan is beneficial for:

- the necessary physiological re-set most people need,
- potentially insulin resistant/pre-diabetics,
- diabetics,
- those experiencing blood sugar, blood pressure, cholesterol issues, etc.,
- inflamed individuals,
- those in pain,
- depressed individuals,
- anxious individuals,
- toxic people,
- the sick who require healing,
- and those who experience seizures.

The Advanced Plan is similar to a low carb diet, but it is not high protein or toxic like many of those diets are. PLUS—it's not all about deprivation. You are simply replacing the carbs with fats, proteins, and all those grain-free, properly sweetened dessert recipes that are so abundant in this plan. It's *Advanced* weight loss—but you still get to eat!

The Core Plan

The Core Plan includes healthy grains and naturally occurring sugars. It's great for kids or individuals who have already reached their ideal weight and just want to be healthy. A young, active person would likely lose weight and/or get super lean while older, more sedentary individuals will be able to maintain their weight. This is an ideal program for marathon preparation and competitive athletes doing intense training.

Weight loss following this plan is particularly attainable if you're only modestly overweight, have put on a few pounds, and/or are not yet experiencing metabolic symptoms like high cholesterol or high blood pressure.

As we mentioned, for many, the idea is to implement the Advanced Plan until you've hit your health and fitness goals, and then add in Core foods.

Advanced Plan is not a "high protein" plan, and the Core Plan isn't high carb. To help moderate your carb intake and keep your protein intake to 20-30 grams per meal, go to Appendix II and III for the Carb Counter and the Protein Counter.

Enjoying the Plans for Life: The Vacation Rule

The purpose of anything I share is to make your life easier, not harder to live than it is right now. You'll have to make some conscious decisions to eat better, and while that may sound impossible—it's very possible, I promise.

A common reflex is to re-sist new diets because it means you never get to enjoy life again. So, let's get acquainted with the "Vacation Rule."

The Vacation idea is simple: having nachos or pizza for lunch once a week and ice cream on Sunday afternoon *isn't going to hurt.* In fact, it might even help you. And when you take that Spring Break vacation, take a couple days off the diet. It's mentally healthy—and in some ways, it's even physically healthy.

What you'll find is that over time, you'll choose more and more healthy vacation options because you feel so good with foods by God and…so bad without them.

Between tasty, healthy recipes and the Vacation Rule, you're go-ing to enjoy this. It's when you don't feel like you're really "sacrificing" that you truly make lasting changes.

7 Basic Rules of Nutrition to Follow

- Eliminate soft drinks, sugar sweetened beverages and any non-fresh juices.
- Eat fruit in the morning and load up on vegetables at all other meals and the rest of the day. (You can load up on vegetables in the morning too if you want to really get fresh, live foods in your body.)
- Switch to good fats: Cook with coconut oil and butter, and put olive oil on salads. Find ways to add chia seeds, flax seeds, and fish from the safe list to your week.
- Dump the candy and sugar-filled desserts. Use fruit or the grain-free, sugar free desserts we give you.
- Do organic meats and dairy as much as possible, and reduce your intake of commercial animal products.
- Eliminate wheat, rye, barley, and baked goods from your diet.
- No fried foods!

The Genesis Food List

The Genesis Food List contains some of the common foods and ingre-dients eaten for breakfast, lunch, dinner, and snacks. For the complete list with explanation, go to Appendix I: *Thou Shall Eat This. Thou Shall not Eat That.*

Breakfast

Advanced Foods

Almond, coconut flour

Avocado

Blackberries

Blueberries

Cheeses (organic recommended)

Chia seed

Coconut milk

Eggs

Flax seed

Goat's milk or organic yogurt

Granny Smith apples

Grass-fed dairy products

Organic butter

Raspberries

Raw nuts*, seeds*, Nut butter (without added oils or sugars)

Smoothies

Stevia

Strawberries

Vegan protein powder: hemp, pea, brown rice

Vegetables

Grass-fed whey powder

Core Foods

Ancient grains*: amaranth, quinoa, and millet

Higher sugar fruits: bananas, grapes, pineapple, red apples, plums, watermelon

Oatmeal (gluten free)

Raw, organic honey, coconut sugar, organic maple syrup

Lunch

Advanced Foods

Almond, coconut flour

Avocado

Berries

Carrots

Cheeses (organic recommended)

Chia seeds

Extra virgin coconut oil

Green smoothies

Legumes* (beans, lentils, peanuts, peas, etc.)

Nut butter (without added oils or sugars)

Raw nuts*, seeds*, and nut flour

Safe fish (see list)

Extra virgin olive oil

Flax seeds

Granny Smith apples

Grapeseed oil dressing

Salads

Steak/beef/chicken
(organic recommended)

Vegetables

Core Foods

Ancient grains*: amaranth, quinoa, and millet

Brown rice

Higher sugar fruits: bananas, grapes, pineapple, red apples,

plums, watermelon

Sweet potato

Dinner

Advanced Foods

Almond, coconut flour

Asparagus

Avocado

Broccoli

Brussels sprouts

Cabbage

Cauliflower

Cheeses
(organic recommended)

Extra virgin coconut oil

Extra virgin olive oil

Safe fish: sardines, tilapia, salmon,
flounder, herring

Salads

Steak/chicken
(organic recommended)

Vegetables

Core Foods

Ancient grains*: amaranth, quinoa, and millet

Brown rice

Legumes*: beans, lentils, peanuts, peas, etc.

Fruit

[*Please see the sprouting instructions for legumes, grains, nuts, and seeds in Appendix IV.]

The Key to Snacks and Desserts

One way to really crave carbs is to get to the point where you're starving and ready to eat a hippo. The key with snacks is to avoid starvation while not adding carbs between meals. If you do an after dinner snack, it should be eaten 2-3 hours before bed – although vegetables are always "free" even right before bedtime. If you're perfectly satisfied or struggling to lose weight, then you don't need to eat between meals or after dinner.

Snack Suggestions

- Granny Smith apple alone or with 1-2 tablespoons almond or peanut butter. Nut butters should have no added ingredients—just the nut

- Celery with 1-2 tablespoons of almond or peanut butter or organic cream cheese

- Vegetable sticks (celery, cucumber, green/red/yellow pepper, Romaine) with yogurt veggie dip,* guacamole, or hummus

- ½ cup of Greek or goat's milk yogurt with Stevia to taste, shredded coconut, shaved unsweetened chocolate, and ground flax seeds or chia seeds

- Green smoothie

- The dessert recipes—remember, they're made of nut flours, good fats, and non-sugar sweeteners so they're a food.

- Mixed sweet nuts*

- Raw almonds, pistachios, peanuts (on occasion), hazelnuts, and pecans. Cashews are higher on the Glycemic index (so only for the more active or on Core Plan)

- Salads and leftover cooked proteins and vegetables

- Chocolate malted smoothie*

- Breakfast recipes like Grain-less Granola* and Brownie Cereal* and dessert recipes like avocado or chia seed pudding* or no-guilt chocolate chip cookies* make for great snacks!

[*See recipes.]

Desserts in our plan provide limited carbs and can be eaten for snacks and after meals. We've placed something sweet after dinner in the plan, but it's not an absolute. Again, if satisfied, it's your choice to partake or not.

Supplement Guide & Guidance

High quality, whole food supplements should make up a part of your regular nutrition plan. You just don't get the nutrients you need for optimum functioning from diet alone. Twenty-five years of practice and analyzing 100s of 1000s of patients has led me and the other doctors I work with to recommend a certain supplement baseline. These include:

1. A daily detoxification supplement

2. Vitamin D

3. An omega fatty acid supplement

4. Women's or men's multivitamin

5. A daily anti-inflammatory supplement

6. A greens product

7. Grass-fed whey or the vegetarian alternative

You can see the supplement planning and dose guideline after the meal plans (page 34).

Some Explanation to the Maximizing Cooking and Meal Plans

One way to cut costs, make it easier, and increase convenience is to cook enough of one meal for 2-3 meals at a time. Then, the next day, you eat the leftovers—which are almost always better the second day—rather than having to cook again.

Leftovers also make great snacks. If you're hungry between meals or after dinner, you can eat leftovers—which you know are safe and fit the plan.

On a tight budget? See the Cost-Cutter Options after the Meal Plan shopping list.

The following meal plans ensure that if you, someone in your family, or someone who cooks for you likes to shop and prepare recipes, you can create great tasting dishes with tons of variety. Or like others, you may simply like the basics for "staple" meals.

Staple Meal Example—My Staple Foods

- Breakfast: eggs, smoothies, or unsweetened yogurt sweetened with Stevia, berries, and other healthy additions.
- Lunch: salads with protein, olive oil dressings, and healthy, raw and/or organic cheeses.
- Snacks: Granny Smith apples, raw nuts and seeds, and grain-free, sugar free desserts.
- Dinner: Chicken/fish/grass-fed meat, salad, and steamed or stir fried vegetables, grain-free, sugar-free dessert.

We've named specific meals, snacks, and dessert examples in the plan (coming up on the next page), but you can choose from the many recipes we've provided that are listed by breakfast, lunch, dinner, or snack. It's all about mixing, matching, and making this plan work for you!

30-Day Challenge Meal Plan

		BREAKFAST	LUNCH	DINNER	SNACK/ DESSERT
WEEK 1					
1	MONDAY	Berry breakfast smoothie	Turkey cheese-burger on Bibb lettuce	Chargrilled chicken, roasted broccoli and baby spinach salad	Chocolate-avocado brownies with walnuts (1)
2	TUESDAY	Spinach and egg omelet	Vegetable kabobs with pesto and char-grilled chicken	Black bean chili	Chocolate-avocado brownies with walnuts (1)
3	WEDNESDAY	Nutrition Knock-Out Green breakfast smoothie	Leftovers: Black bean chili	Broiled tilapia and steamed veggies	Celery sticks with 1-2 tablespoons almond or peanut butter, or organic cream cheese
4	THURSDAY	Scrambled eggs with apple	Broiled tilapia over a mixed green and macadamia nut salad	Spiced steak with grilled pepper salad	Crispy butterscotch cookies (2)
5	FRIDAY	"Kitchen-sink" yogurt	Romaine and avocado salad with spiced steak strips	Mediterranean stew	Crispy butterscotch cookies (2)

	BREAKFAST	LUNCH	DINNER	SNACK/DESSERT
WEEK 1				
6 SATURDAY	Fried eggs and cherry tomatoes	Leftovers: Mediterranean stew	Baked basil chicken over fresh greens with asparagus	Cinnamon almonds (½ cup)
7 SUNDAY	2 eggs and an avocado	Spinach and toasted walnut salad with baked chicken	Grilled salmon, zucchini, and broccoli salad	Gooey chocolate chip cookies (2)

30-Day Challenge Meal Plan: *Week 2*

	BREAKFAST	LUNCH	DINNER	SNACK/DESSERT
WEEK 2				
8 MONDAY	Scrambled Eggs with Apple	Grilled Salmon Salad with Blueberries and Mint	Steak and Asparagus Stir-Fry	Gooey Chocolate Chip Cookies (2)
9 TUESDAY	Chocolate-Covered Strawberry Smoothie	LEFTOVERS: Steak and Asparagus Stir-Fry	Baked Chicken and Sautéed Brussels Sprouts	Vegetable Sticks Veggie Yogurt Dip
10 WEDNESDAY	"Kitchen-sink" yogurt	Turkey Cheese Burger on Bibb Lettuce	Barbecued Sirloin in Dijon Dressing with Grilled Vegetables	Chocolate-Avocado Brownies with Walnuts (1)
11 THURSDAY	2 Eggs and Fresh Berries	Leftovers: Barbecued Sirloin in Dijon Dressing with Grilled Vegetables	Chargrilled Chicken and Roasted Broccoli and Baby Spinach Salad	Chocolate-Avocado Brownies with Walnuts (1)
12 FRIDAY	Spinach and Egg Omelet	Chargrilled Chicken, Blackberry and Baby Arugula Salad	Mediterranean stew	Almond Butter "Granola" Bars
13 SATURDAY	Cherry Vanilla Green Smoothie	Leftovers: Mediterranean stew	Broiled Tilapia and Steamed Veggies	Almond Butter "Granola" Bars
14 SUNDAY	"Kitchen-sink" yogurt	Vegetable Ratatouille	Black Bean Chili	4-5 Celery Sticks filled with Almond or Peanut Butter

30-Day Challenge Meal Plan: *Week 3*

		BREAKFAST	LUNCH	DINNER	SNACK/DESSERT
WEEK 3					
15	MONDAY	Nutrition knock-out green breakfast smoothie	Leftovers: black bean chili	Spiced steak and grilled pepper salad	Chocolate-dipped macaroons
16	TUESDAY	2 eggs and fresh berries	Strawberry, romaine, and avocado salad with spiced steak strips	Grilled salmon, zucchini, and broccoli salad	Chocolate-dipped macaroons
17	WEDNESDAY	Chocolate-covered strawberry smoothie	Turkey Cheese Burger on Bibb Lettuce	Steak and asparagus stir-fry	Cinnamon almonds (½ cup)
18	THURSDAY	Fried eggs and cherry tomatoes	Leftovers: steak and asparagus stir-fry	Chargrilled Chicken and Roasted Broccoli and Baby Spinach Salad	Crispy butterscotch cookies (2)
19	FRIDAY	"Kitchen sink" yogurt	Char-grilled chicken salad with white beets	Grilled salmon, zucchini and broccoli salad	Crispy butterscotch cookies (2)
20	SATURDAY	Vegetable and egg breakfast scramble	Vegetable ratatouille	Mediterranean stew	Celery sticks with 1-2 tablespoons almond or peanut butter, or organic cream cheese
21	SUNDAY	Strawberries and spinach green smoothie	Leftovers: Mediterranean stew	Barbecued sirloin in Dijon dressing with grilled vegetables	Gooey chocolate chip cookies (2)

30-Day Challenge Meal Plan: *Week 4*

		BREAKFAST	LUNCH	DINNER	SNACK/DESSERT
WEEK 4					
22	MONDAY	Spinach and egg omelet	Leftovers: barbecued sirloin in Dijon dressing with grilled vegetables	Char-grilled chicken, roasted broccoli, and baby spinach salad	Gooey chocolate chip cookies (2)
23	TUESDAY	"Kitchen sink" yogurt	Turkey cheese-burger on Bibb lettuce	Mediterranean stew	Cinnamon almonds (½ cup)

	BREAKFAST	LUNCH	DINNER	SNACK/ DESSERT
WEEK 4				
24 WEDNESDAY	Berry breakfast smoothie	Leftovers: Mediterranean stew	Baked chicken and sautéed Brussels sprouts	Crispy butterscotch cookies
25 THURSDAY	Fried eggs and cherry tomatoes	Vegetable ratatouille	Broiled tilapia and steamed veggies	Crispy butterscotch cookies (2)
26 FRIDAY	Cherry and vanilla green smoothie	Mixed greens and tilapia salad with macadamia nuts	Black bean chili	Vegetable sticks Veggie Yogurt Dip
27 SATURDAY	2 eggs and fresh berries	Leftover: black bean chili	Char-grilled chicken and roasted broccoli	Almond butter "granola" bars
28 SUNDAY	Nutrition knock-out green breakfast smoothie	Grilled chicken chopped salad	Spiced steak and grilled pepper salad	Almond butter "granola" bars

30-Day Challenge Meal Plan: *Week 5*

	BREAKFAST	LUNCH	DINNER	SNACK/ DESSERT
WEEK 5				
29 MONDAY	Chocolate-covered strawberry smoothie	Vegetable kabobs with pesto	Mediterranean stew	Celery sticks with 1-2 tablespoons almond or peanut butter, or organic cream cheese
30 TUESDAY	Spinach and egg omelet	Leftovers: Mediterranean stew	Steak and asparagus stir-fry	Chocolate-dipped macaroons

[*See additional cost cutter recipes in the recipe section starting on page 71.]

The Maximized Living Supplementation Plan

Detox System® (Cell Detox + Body Detox) is a unique two part system. It starts with Cell Detox, which provides a whole foods formula that contains traditional natural detoxifying herbs, amino acids, probiotics and antioxidants that support you all the way down to the cellular level. Body Detox provides whole food magnesium and fiber, traditional botanicals and activated charcoal for healthy elimination.

- Detoxification is contingent upon healthy glutathione levels which are supported by Cysteine, Glycine and Glutamine.
- Activated charcoal, flax seed and psyllium husk bind to toxins and support healthy elimination.
- Milk Thistle and sulphur purify the liver while peppermint leaf and ginger soothe the digestive tract.

Vitamin D3 Complex® is Maximized Living's Vitamin D3 formula containing 1000 IU of Vitamin D3 which helps support immune health, healthy bones, joint, digestive health, skin and teeth. This formula is free of additives like gluten, yeast, dairy, sugar, starch or artificial coloring, making it a superior product.

- A complex cultivated within 22 organic fruits and vegetables including superfoods like broccoli, kale and spinach to facilitate superior absorption
- Probiotic support with Bacillus coagulans, for healthy digestion, improved metabolism and normal immune response.
- 5000 IU of Vitamin D in one convenient capsule.

Max Fit® is a multidimensional, whole food formula to maintain healthy weight, energy and metabolism. This formula supports stress management and cortisol regulation to improve energy and vitality. Make the most of your workout by adding Max Fit to the mix!

- A superior blend of glutamine, carnitine and creatine support healthy metabolism.
- Powerful Ashwaganda improves energy, endurance and power while supporting cortisol regulation.

- Decaffeinated green coffee bean extract supports healthy blood glucose levels and supports healthy weight when combined with diet and exercise.

Perfect Plant Protein® is packed full of essential amino acids, fiber, supreme doses of vitamins and trace minerals. Perfect Plant Protein is the ideal product to help maintain healthy energy levels and optimal nutrition. In the hustle and bustle of everyday life, it is challenging to get enough of what we need: sleep, exercise, water and relaxation. Our Perfect Plant Protein contains essential amino acids formed by over a dozen sprouted grains, seeds and beans. The sprouted brown rice in this unique formula contains an abundance of nutrients—more than cooked brown rice!

- Promotes lean muscle and stimulates fat loss while stabilizing blood sugar levels.
- Provides energy, boosts immunity, repairs muscle and supports healthy bones.
- Defends the body against free radical damage and toxins.

Max Greens® is a unique formulation that features 34 organic and living super foods. This highly digestible formula is full of greens, veggie juices and sprouts that are rich in chlorophyll, antioxidants and trace minerals. Max Greens boosts energy, facilitates detoxification and supports maximized digestion through enzymes and probiotics! It's time to help your body live more healthfully! Max Greens is ideal for vegans, vegetarians, athletes, and anyone who needs a veggie boost on the go.

- Garlic, ginger and beet combine to provide organ cleansing and detoxification support.
- Superior probiotic support with Saccharomyces boulardii, a strain shown to support healthy immune response, reduced inflammation and improved digestive function.
- Mineral rich broccoli, kale and spinach provide antioxidants and improved energy.

Men's Multi® is a formula with specialized nutrients and vitamins to support prostate, bone, heart, skin and reproductive health. Our whole foods based multivitamin provides essential vitamins, minerals, probiotics and enzymes using 18 different fruits and vegetables. As an added benefit, our formula contains a specialized muscle recovery blend, digestive support and immune support.

- Probiotic support with Lactobacillus plantarum, a strain shown to promote normal digestion, destroy pathogens and preserve critical nutrients, vitamins and antioxidants.

- Antioxidant support through kelp, spinach and powerful mixed tocopherols.

- Maximized Vitamin C blend with amla and grapefruit bioflavonoids to provide a super immune boost.

Women's Multi® is a formula with specialized nutrients and vitamins to support breast, bone, heart, skin and reproductive health. Our whole foods based multivitamin provides essential vitamins, minerals, probiotics and enzymes using 18 different fruits and vegetables. As an added benefit, our formula contains a specialized women's wellness blend, bioflavonoids and antioxidants.

- Probiotic support with Lactobacillus plantarum, a strain shown to promote normal digestion, destroy pathogens and preserve critical nutrients, vitamins and antioxidants.

- Antioxidant support through kelp, spinach and powerful mixed tocopherols.

- Maximized wellness blend that supports healthy stress management and naturally addresses inflammation.

Optimal Omega® is a formula developed to provide essential fatty acids in ratios that promote a healthy lifestyle. Omegas provide the fatty acids necessary for optimal cardiovascular and circulatory health, healthy immune response, healthy skin and eyes, and improved cognitive function.

- 2400mg of ultra-pure and highly effective Omega 3 and Omega 6.

- Also includes 160mg of GLA, which helps reduce inflammation.

- 10 IU (33% of DV) of Vitamin E for antioxidant support.

Perfect Protein® is derived from 100% naturally raised cows. Never injected with hormones, fed grains or genetically modified foods, our cows graze on natural grass pastures free of pesticides and chemicals. Vital enzymes, probiotics, immune factors, and amino acids remain intact through low-temperature, delicate filtration to prevent any nutrient damage. Our protein promotes lean muscle and stimulates fat loss while stabilizing blood sugar levels, boosting energy and immunity and supporting bone health. ML Perfect Protein is the ideal protein powder for your everyday health or for enhanced recovery from exercise.

- Fortified with vitamins and minerals, plus Glucosamine for collagen and cartilage strength.
- Packed with Lysine, an essential amino acid that plays a role in weight management and bone health by working synergistically with magnesium and calcium.
- 20 grams of protein per serving to fuel your body and support optimal health.

Daily Defense® is a whole foods formulation that provides a powerful combination of 3 synergistic antioxidants: turmeric, Indian gooseberry and cantaloupe extract. This powerful trio of antioxidants combats free radical damage and oxidative stress and supports healthy aging and regeneration. Give your body what it needs to combat oxidative stress and free radical damage and you'll experience a healthier immune system, less pain and improved systemic function.

- Contains a patented form of curcumin known as C3 Complex. The name C3 Complex has reference to the three main compounds found in curcumin: Curcumin, Demethoxycurcumin and Bisdemethoxycurcumin. Curcumin has antioxidant, antimicrobial, and anticancer properties.
- Indian Gooseberry is another powerful antioxidant that has been studied for its ability to heal and possibly prevent atherosclerosis and heart disease.
- Melon extract is a source of Superoxide Dismutase (SOD), a potent antioxidant that fights cellular damage.

Max GI® is a digestive support formula that contains enzymes, probiotics, essential oils and minerals designed to balance the GI tract and repair intestinal permeability. Our formula provides a targeted solution to support proper gastrointestinal function, necessary for the effective elimination of toxins and healthy immune system performance. Be your best self with clinical strength digestive support!

- Lysozyme provides protection from bacteria by breaking down bacterial cell walls.
- Probiotic support with bacillus subtillis, an organism that stimulates the immune system and prevents bacteria and viruses from crossing the gut lining.
- Essential oils of Clove, Oregano and Thyme defend against bacterial invasions and support a strong and healthy immune system.

When and How to Take Each:

Time of Day	Supplement	Dose
MORNING: 30 MINUTES BEFORE BREAKFAST	• Cell Detox • Max Fit	• 2 capsules • 1 capsule
MORNING: 15 MINUTES BEFORE BREAKFAST	• Max GI	• 2 capsules
MORNING: WITH MEAL	• Women's/Men's Multi- Optimal Omega • Daily Defense • Vitamin D3 Complex • Max Greens • Perfect Protein • Perfect Plant Protein	• 2 capsules • 1 softgel • 1 capsule • 1 capsule • 1 scoop • 1 scoop • 1 scoop
BETWEEN BREAKFAST AND LUNCH: 30 MINUTES BEFORE LUNCH	• Max Fit	• 1 capsule
WITH LUNCH:	• Optimal Omega	• 1 softgel
BETWEEN LUNCH AND DINNER: 30 MINUTES BEFORE DINNER	• Max Fit	• 1 capsule
ONE HOUR BEFORE BEDTIME:	• Body Detox	• 2 capsules

MDS® (Maximized Delivery System): A proprietary nutrient-dense matrix of whole food ingredients to give you increased absorption, utilization and potency.

To order these supplements, visit your Maximized Living Doctor's website. If you don't have one, find one near you at maximizedliving.com or shop at store.maximizedliving.com

30-Day Meal Plan: The Grocery List

With all these yummy recipes, you're probably going to need to add some supplies to your stock. But no need to get overwhelmed making a list... because we've already made one for you! Simply take this along with you to grocery shop, and you're all set!

Produce & Fresh Herbs

- ☐ Apples, Granny Smith—10
  (Organic when possible; on Environmental Working Groups [EWG} s 2014's Dirty Dozen List)
- ☐ Asparagus—2 lbs.
- ☐ Avocados—5
- ☐ Baby Arugula—1-2 bunches (5 cups)
- ☐ Baby Carrots—5 cups
- ☐ Baby Spinach—1-2 bunches (8 cups)
  (Organic when possible; on EWG's 2014's Dirty Dozen List)
- ☐ Bell Pepper, Green—2 *(Organic when possible; on EWG's 2014's Dirty Dozen List)*
- ☐ Bell Pepper, Red—3 *(Organic when possible; on EWG's 2014's Dirty Dozen List)*
- ☐ Boston Lettuce—1 Head (or Bibb Lettuce, if preferred)
- ☐ Broccoli—1 bunch
- ☐ Brussels Sprouts
- ☐ Cauliflower—1 head
- ☐ Celery—2 Bunches *(Organic when possible; on EWG's 2014's Dirty Dozen List)*
- ☐ Cherry Tomatoes—3 pints
  (Organic when possible; on EWG's 2014's Dirty Dozen List)
- ☐ Cucumber—2 *(Organic when possible; on EWG's 2014's Dirty Dozen List)*
- ☐ Eggplants—3
- ☐ Fresh Basil—1 small bunch
- ☐ Fresh Berries (of choice)—3.5 pints (7 cups)
- ☐ Fresh Blackberries—2 pints (4 cups)
- ☐ Fresh Flat-Leaf Parsley—1 bunch
- ☐ Fresh Garlic—2 bulbs
- ☐ Fresh Ginger—1 small piece
- ☐ Fresh Lemons—1 bag
- ☐ Fresh Limes—4 limes
- ☐ Fresh Mixed Greens (of choice)—4 cups
- ☐ Fresh Strawberries—5 pints (10 cups)
  (Organic when possible; on EWG's 2014's Dirty Dozen List)
- ☐ Green Onions—1 small bunch
- ☐ Jicama—2
- ☐ Kale—2-3 bunches of choice (18 cups)
  (Organic when possible; on EWG's 2014's Dirty Dozen List)
- ☐ Large, Ripe Tomatoes—4
- ☐ Lemongrass—1 small bunch
- ☐ Mixed Vegetables of Choice—8 cups
- ☐ Onion, Yellow—1

- ☐ Onions, White—3
- ☐ Onions, Red—2
- ☐ Raw Spinach—2 bunches (10 cups)
  (Organic when possible; on EWG's 2014's Dirty Dozen List)
- ☐ Romaine Lettuce—1 head (6 cups)
- ☐ Spirulina—1 small bunch
- ☐ Water Chestnuts—1 can
- ☐ White Beets
- ☐ Zucchini—6 large

Proteins—Meats, Eggs, Nuts & Seeds

- ☐ Flax Seeds and/or Chia Seeds – ½ cup
- ☐ Free-Range Boneless Skinless Chicken Breasts = 8 *(6 oz. each fillets)*
- ☐ Grass-Fed Sirloin Steaks, New York Cut – 4 (4-6 oz. each) steaks
- ☐ Grass-Fed Sirloin Steaks, preferred cut – 9 (4-6 oz. each) steaks
- ☐ Pasture-Raised Eggs, Large = 23
- ☐ Pistachio Nuts – ¼ cup
- ☐ Raw Sliced Almonds – smallest package you can find
  (if buying in bulk – you only need 2 tablespoons.)
- ☐ Sesame Seeds – ¼ cup
- ☐ Walnuts – 2 cup
- ☐ Wild-Caught Salmon – 2 (6 oz.) fillets
- ☐ Tilapia Fillets –3 (4-6 oz.) fillets
- ☐ Pecans
- ☐ Macadamia Nuts

Pantry, Baking Needs & Miscellaneous Items

- ☐ 6 Bamboo Skewers
- ☐ 10 oz. Enjoy Life vegan dark chocolate (or semisweet chocolate)
- ☐ Almond Butter – 1-2 containers (or Peanut Butter)
- ☐ Almond Flour – 3 cups
- ☐ Baking Powder
- ☐ Baking Soda
- ☐ Beef Broth – 1 can
- ☐ Chicken Broth, Reduced Sodium – 3 cans
- ☐ Chocolate Perfect Protein Powder – 1 scoop
- ☐ Coconut Aminos
- ☐ Coconut Cream – 2 cans

- ☐ Coconut Flour – 1 cup
- ☐ Coconut Milk – 3 cans
- ☐ Coconut Oil
- ☐ Coconut Water – 1 can/bottle (optional – for smoothies – can also use filtered water)
- ☐ Dijon Mustard
- ☐ Extra Virgin Olive Oil
- ☐ Gluten-Free Cannellini Beans – 2 to 3 cans
- ☐ Preferred Hummus – ½ cup
- ☐ Preferred Pesto Sauce – 1 jar
- ☐ Stevia Powder Extract and/or Stevia Packets
- ☐ Sun-Dried Tomatoes – 1 jar
- ☐ Tapioca Starch
- ☐ Unsweetened Cocoa Powder
- ☐ Unsweetened Organic All-Natural Applesauce – ½ cup
- ☐ Unsweetened, Shredded Coconut – 1 package
- ☐ Vanilla Perfect Protein Powder – 4 scoops
- ☐ Vegan Chocolate Chips (such as Enjoy Life) – 1 package
- ☐ Vegan Mayonnaise (Such as Hellmann's)
- ☐ Vegetable Broth – 5 cans
- ☐ Vinegar – Apple Cider Vinegar
- ☐ Vinegar – Balsamic Vinegar
- ☐ Vinegar – White Wine Vinegar
- ☐ Xylitol

Spices, Seasonings & Extracts

- ☐ Cayenne Pepper
- ☐ Butterscotch Extract
- ☐ Chili Powder
- ☐ Crushed Red Pepper Flakes
- ☐ Curry Powder
- ☐ Dried Parsley
- ☐ Fresh Ground Black Pepper
- ☐ Ground Cinnamon
- ☐ Ground Coriander
- ☐ Ground Cumin
- ☐ Ground Flaxseed
- ☐ Ground Nutmeg

☐	Sea Salt
☐	Tarragon
☐	Vanilla Extract
☐	White Pepper

Refrigerated & Frozen Items

☐	Frozen Cherries, Organic; Pitted – 1 package
☐	Grass-Fed Butter – 8 oz. Package
☐	Organic Whole (or Goat's Milk) Plain Yogurt – 2 pints

Run For Hope:
Take the Challenge—Even If You're Coming Off the Couch!

If you want to become the best runner you can be, start now. Don't spend the rest of your life wondering if you can do it. —Priscilla Welch
(Quit smoking at 35, made the 1984 Olympics 4 years later, and won the 1987 NY Marathon)

I'm not what I ought to be, I'm not what I want to be, But I'm better than I used to be. And I'm not what I'm going to be. —Old Country Prayer)

Scheduling a race: we call this *"a smart move."* Having a race to get ready for is the most impactful way to make a long-term commitment to exercise! So, set a race date! Whether you're coming off the couch or already a runner, this program is specifically designed to help you attain an optimal level of fitness to successfully complete a 5K race in just 6 weeks, a 10K in 8 weeks, a Half-Marathon in 12 weeks, or a Marathon in just 16 weeks!

Don't be intimidated. Just start nice and easy and build up. In addition to making this easier to complete, we'll help you build up your training volume and intensity gradually over the course of several weeks, which is beneficial for maximum performance, injury prevention, and avoiding burning out.

Everything you need is laid out for you from nutrition to supplementation to fitness regimens and more. You will be surprised at just how much your body can accomplish in the period of just 6, 8, 12, or 16 weeks!

Remember: It is important to always consult with your physician before taking on this or any new nutrition/fitness regimen.

Understanding the Runs

In the training programs, you'll see:

1. *Run/walk:* Pick a manageable time or distance and then do a 1-2 minute recovery walk and repeat. Do this for the length of the required time or distance that day.

2. *Easy run:* Known also as a "recovery run." This is a comfortable jogging pace.

3. *Run:* Stay in a zone where you can still talk with a running partner but going at a pace above jogging. Choose a pace that you believe is sustainable for the entire workout.

Enhancing Performance

1. *Tempo:* this this is a pace at or just below racing level. Sustaining this for a pre-determined amount of minutes or a whole run will add enormous value to your race preparation.

2. *Intervals:* Any walk or run can be enhanced by short surges of higher intensity walks or runs to increase heart rate followed by slower recovery phases before more high intensity surges. This method can be sprinkled into any walk or run, is proven to increase performance more than any other method and is highly encouraged especially as someone gets fitter.

For Longer Runs

Longer runs require a slower pace. As you get in better and better shape, the tendency may be to speed up at the beginning, and pay for it at the end by not being able to finish or finish well. It's always best to start slower, and pick it up at the end if you're feeling good.

Your Secret Weapon: MaxT3

Making exercise 10X more effective in 1/10th the time

One-to-two times per week, the training plans recommend the following MaxT3 workout. These MaxT3 days turn you into a fat-burning, muscle-building machine. They exponentially change body composition and improve the function of your metabolic engine, so you can better perform, run, and just live life.

T3 equals time, type, and tempo (intensity level). On the days you utilize these plans, you'll optimize all 3 of these T's. This is done by directly impacting your muscle to fat ratio as well as boosting the good hormones that cause you to be the kind of person you most likely hate—someone who naturally tends to be thin, lean, and in shape!

The secret to the results is high-tempo, short-time—as opposed to the typical long, low intensity runs and workouts most people perform when getting ready for a race.

These workouts show you how to easily leverage time, tempo, and type to your advantage, and they're incredibly safe as you perform at personally achievable maximum levels.

These are superior workouts for all types. A beginner can use this to get in shape, and we can adapt this for Olympians, professional athletes, and those striving to compete at the highest level.

How to Perform MaxT3

In high-tempo, short-duration exercise, you go as fast as you physically can, and do exercises designed to really push your system for brief periods, followed by enough recovery time so you can repeat.

With high-intensity, short-duration exercise, your body *responds* by increasing the hormones and physiology you need to burn fat and produce muscle. As a result, you not only build muscle and burn fat *during* exercise, but your body does so for hours after.

Additionally, the more muscle you have, the more tendency there is to produce *more* muscle. It's muscle and not age, gender, or genetics that is the greatest determining factor for metabolism and future muscle development.

The MaxT3 Training Plan

These consist of intermittent bursts or surges you can only maintain for a short time period. You give maximum output for a designated time, distance, or exercise. Then, you recover during the prescribed time enough to allow your heart rate to reset, and then you surge again.

There are a multitude of ways to combine the cardio and resistance aspects of MaxT3 that offer a ton of variety, so you never get bored. With exercise, variety really is the spice of life. We vary the exercises, so we address all aspects of fitness—core, flexibility, balance, strength, muscle building, and fat burning.

Important for Beginners and Intermediates

It's very important to modify the exercises to match your level of conditioning. For example: if the move is a push-up, you can also do the push-ups from your knees instead of your feet. If the move is a squat, you can hang onto a chair to keep the pressure on your knees and legs extremely light. If the exercise calls for resistance, you can use something as light as a soup can, a book, or a light dumbbell. Listen to your body. This is your workout!

Important for everyone: I highly recommend you get the MaxT3 videos (www.MaxT3.com). You'll see that we've added 1-2 MaxT3 days to your training schedule in the Run for Hope plans. It is, however, difficult to write about exercise and put on paper enough variety to keep you interested long term and maximize your results.

The Monday MaxT3 Workout

Looking through each fitness regimen, you will see the term "Max T3" on Mondays. Again, this will be your secret-weapon fitness tool in this program to help get your body into optimum shape for your race.

Before starting, find your training heart rate through the following calculations:

- 220 minus (–) your age = your maximum heart rate
- 75 to 85% of your maximum heart rate is your training heart rate.

Experienced athletes can go beyond this number. Subtract 10 if you're a beginner or experiencing or recovering from health problems. Stop the workout if you're not an elite athlete and your heart rate reaches 100 percent or more of your training heart rate. Remember to always consult a physician before starting any new exercise program.

MaxT3 Exertion & Workout Guidelines

- All rounds should be completed as fast as possible while pushing the intensity throughout the entire workout. The exception is when just beginning the program or if contending with an injury.

- Make sure you get enough rest between rounds to be able to go all out. You lose the power of MaxT3 if you're too tired and go slow—then it's just jogging.

- Rest times between sprints or hard runs are 60-120 seconds.

- *Important for beginners and intermediates:* it's very important to modify the exercises to your level of conditioning.

MaxT3 Run Exertion Explanation

- Jog: A relaxed, slow, comfortable pace to warm up.

- Sprint: Only able to sustain the pace for 50-100 meters.

- Sprint-Run: Start out sprinting as far as you can, backing down to a pace more manageable for you to finish the distance or time.

- Cross Training: Cross Training days mean that you add non-running cardio exercise in like swimming, biking, elliptical, etc. for 20 minutes to an hour.

- Off-day Options: You get two off-days a week and want to completely rest your legs on those days. However, for one of your off days, it's great to build up your core and upper body strength. Once again, it's recommend you get the MaxT3 video, and add the core and upper body routines. They're over in 12 minutes (so like a day off) but make a radical difference in your shape, fitness, and running. www.maxt3.com

5K/10K/Half-Marathon/Marathon Program Success Tips

These daily and weekly guidelines will assist you in effectively keeping track of your progress throughout the course of your program.

You learn you can do your best even when it's hard, even when you're tired and maybe hurting a little bit. It feels good to show some courage.
—Joe Namath

Have I not commanded you? Be strong and courageous. Do not be afraid; do not be discouraged, for the LORD your God will be with you wherever you go.
—Joshua 1:9

DAILY GUIDELINES	WEEKLY GUIDELINES
Drink During Exercise. Get hand or waist bottle holders, just get used to holding bottles, or plant them along the course of your run.	Track and log your body measurements and use the body measurement log for tracking your progress. Body measurements and not weight is the best (and most accurate) way to check how you're doing.
Be sure to take any supplements recommended by the program for optimum results.	The MaxT3 days are your secret weapon in the plan for getting better results, quicker, and reviving fitness levels beyond what you'd expect for the minimal time that it takes.
Use Advanced and Core foods from the Genesis Food Lists	The Weekly Selfie: Taking a picture of yourself once per week will help you to visually track your progress. You will be able to "see" the changes as they are happening to your body and you will have "Before" and "After" pictures to help keep you motivated and on the right track!
Follow the fitness regimen as designed—pushing yourself too hard too fast can lead to workout burnout and possible injury. If you're more experienced, start the program at a later week point.	Keep a Motivation Journal: Use the journal to jot down your progress, thoughts, and feelings, as well as any goals, inspirational quotes, etc. at least once per week. (Ideally, you'll use your journal more often, but aim for at least once per week!)
Be sure to properly warm up and stretch before and after workouts. Yes, it's an extra 5-10 minutes, but you get to avoid injuries and do this for years as a result.	Keep Your Eye on the Prize: Remind yourself often of your reasons for doing this program, and keep your focus pointed on the finish line. You can use a reward system for completing weekly milestones. This is an excellent way to stay motivated. With each completed week, reward yourself with small items, such as a new CD, a new pair of shoes, a movie night, a mani-pedi, tickets to a game, a vacation meal, etc.

BODY MEASUREMENT LOG

YEAR:

		WEEK 1	WEEK 2	WEEK 3	WEEK 4	WEEK 5	WEEK 6
CHEST	Measure under your arms as high as the tape will go. Keep the tape in a straight line as you bring it around your back.						
UPPER ARMS	Measure wherever biggest above the elbows. (Write one measurement for each upper arm).	Rt: Lt:	Rt: Lt:	Rt: Lt:	Rt: Lt:	Rt: Lt:	Rt: Lt:
WAIST	Your "natural waist" can be found 2-inches above your hipbones. Measure all the way around.						
HIPS	When standing, press legs together and measure at the widest point of your bottom, bring the tapeall the way around.						
THIGHS	Spread your legs while standing; measure all the way around at the biggest part of your thigh. (Write one measurement for each thigh).	Rt: Lt:	Rt: Lt:	Rt: Lt:	Rt: Lt:	Rt: Lt:	Rt: Lt:

Nutrition Recommendation and Training Programs for a 5K, 10K, Half-Marathon, or Marathon

Special Nutritional Considerations for a 5K

- Best recovery meal is to follow one of our smoothie recipes consisting of ingredients like berries, coconut milk, and organic/grass-fed whey protein.

- Hydrating for workouts greater than 30 minutes: drink coconut water following or during exercise greater than 30 minutes.
- Follow the supplement program as recommended.

Special Nutritional Considerations for a 10K

- Drink coconut water for hydration during exercise greater than 30 minutes.
- Best recovery meal is to follow one of our smoothie recipes consisting of ingredients like berries, coconut milk, and organic/grass-fed whey protein.
- Follow the supplement program as recommended.

Special Nutritional Considerations for a Half-Marathon

- Drink coconut water for hydration during exercise.
- Best recovery meal is to follow one of our smoothie recipes consisting of ingredients like berries, coconut milk, and organic/grass-fed whey protein.
- You can also incorporate Core Plan carbs from the Genesis Foods List like higher sugar fruits, sweet potatoes, brown rice, and oatmeal after workouts as well (but not on non-workout days).
- After workouts greater than an hour, you can add in foods with natural sweeteners like raw honey or coconut sugar.
- Follow the supplement program as recommended, but take two additional Daily Defense vitamins on days of runs of 6 miles or more.

Special Nutritional Considerations for a Marathon

- Drink coconut water during and after exercise.
- For runs lasting more than one hour, you need to re-fuel. You have to use what you can stomach and feel good eating. Recommended would be all fruit or fruit sweetened bars if you can eat fruit chews. If choosing gels or other types of endurance fuels, look for those that are honey or fruit sweetened instead of sugar, maltodextrin, corn syrup, and other sweeteners.
- Best recovery meal is to follow one of our smoothie recipes consisting of ingredients like berries, coconut milk, and organic/grass-fed whey protein.

- Add Core Plan foods from the Genesis Foods list like higher sugar fruits, sweet potatoes, brown rice, and oatmeal after workouts and throughout the day.
- After workouts greater than an hour, you can add in foods with natural sweeteners like raw honey or coconut sugar.
- Follow the supplement program as recommended, but take two additional Daily Defense vitamins on days of runs of 6 miles or more.

Finish Your Race!

...and let us run with endurance the race that is set before us, fixing our eyes on Jesus, the author and perfecter of faith, who for the joy set before Him endured the cross, despising the shame, and has sat down at the right hand of the throne of God. —Hebrews 12:1-2

For any training program, if you're already in running shape, jump ahead to later weeks (e.g., 4th or 5th week). If coming off the couch—just start at the beginning, and stay encouraged.

6 WEEKS TO 5K: THE FITNESS PLAN		
WEEK 1		
DAY 1: MONDAY	*MaxT3*	• Warm-up: 10 minute walk/jog • 4 rounds (1 minute rest between each set): 15 Tuck Jumps; 50 meters run-sprint at 90-100% effort; 20 Push-ups; Rest and Repeat
DAY 2: TUESDAY		• Walk 30 minutes
DAY 3: WEDNESDAY		• Walk quickly for 1 mile. Run for 2 minutes or walk quickly for 5 minutes. Keep it up for 1.5 miles (2.5 miles total)
DAY 4: THURSDAY		• OFF (Or MaxT3 Core or Upper Training)
DAY 5: FRIDAY		• Walk 2 miles
DAY 6: SATURDAY		• Run for 2 minutes/walk quickly for 5 minutes for 1.5 miles
DAY 7: SUNDAY		• OFF

WEEK 2		
DAY 8: MONDAY	*MaxT3*	• Warm-up: 10 minute walk/jog • 2 rounds of (1 minute rest between each set): 10 Burpees; 15 Push-ups; 25 Crunches; 10 Jump Squats; 100 meters run-sprint at 90-100% effort; Rest and Repeat
DAY 9: TUESDAY		• Walk 35 minutes
DAY 10: WEDNESDAY		• Walk quickly for 1 mile. Run for 3 minutes or walk quickly for 5 minutes. Keep it up for 2 miles (3 miles total)
DAY 11: THURSDAY		• OFF (Or MaxT3 Core or Upper Training)
DAY 12: FRIDAY		• Run for 3 minutes/walk for 5 minutes for 3 miles
DAY 13: SATURDAY		• Walk 1 mile and then walk/run for 1.5 miles (run 30 seconds; walk 1 minute)
DAY 14: SUNDAY		• OFF

WEEK 3		
DAY 15: MONDAY	*MaxT3*	• Warm-up: Jog ½ mile • 2 rounds each of: 10 Squat Jumps; 15 Shin Slaps; 30 Mountain Climbers; 10 Burpees; Rest and Repeat (2 minutes rest between each set) • 3x100 meter Sprint-Run at 90-100% effort (Rest 60-90 seconds between each set); Rest 2 minutes. • Repeat 3x100 meter Run
DAY 16: TUESDAY		• Walk 3 miles
DAY 17: WEDNESDAY		• Walk quickly for 1 mile. Run for 10 minutes or walk quickly for 5 minutes for 2 miles (3 miles total)
DAY 18: THURSDAY		• OFF (Or MaxT3 Core or Upper Training)
DAY 19: FRIDAY		• CROSS TRAIN DAY: Walk 3 miles or bike/swim/elliptical/rollerblade for 20 minutes
DAY 20: SATURDAY		• Walk 1 mile and run 10 minutes or walk 5 minutes for 2 miles (4 miles total)
DAY 21: SUNDAY		• OFF

WEEK 4

DAY 22: MONDAY	*MaxT3*	• Warm-up: Jog ½ mile • 2 rounds each of: 10 Burpees; 25 Squat Jacks; 15 Diamond Push-ups; 20 Bodyweight Squats; Rest and Repeat (2 minutes rest between each set) • 4x100m Sprint-Run at 90-100% effort. Rest 2 minutes. Repeat (Rest 60-90 seconds between every 2 rounds)
DAY 23: TUESDAY		• Walk 3.5 miles
DAY 24: WEDNESDAY		• Walk quickly for 1 mile. Run for 10 minutes or walk quickly for 5 minutes for 2.5 miles (3.5 miles total)
DAY 25: THURSDAY		• OFF (Or MaxT3 Core or Upper Training)
DAY 26: FRIDAY		• CROSS TRAIN DAY: Walk 3.5 miles or bike/swim/elliptical/ rollerblade for 30 minutes
DAY 27: SATURDAY		• Walk 1 mile and run 10 minutes or walk 5 minutes for 2.5 miles (3.5 miles total)
DAY 28: SUNDAY		• OFF

WEEK 5

DAY 29: MONDAY	*MaxT3*	• Warm-up: Jog 1 mile • 100 Squat Jumps (5 minute limit); Rest 2 minutes • 3x200m Sprint-Run. Rest and Repeat (1-2 minutes rest between each set)
DAY 30: TUESDAY		• Walk 60 minutes
DAY 31: WEDNESDAY		• Walk quickly for 1 mile. Run for 3 minutes or walk for 2 minutes for 3 miles (4 miles total)
DAY 32: THURSDAY		• OFF (Or MaxT3 Core or Upper Training)
DAY 33: FRIDAY		• CROSS TRAIN DAY: 60 minutes or bike/swim/elliptical/ rollerblade for 45 minutes
DAY 34: SATURDAY		• Run for 3 miles
DAY 35: SUNDAY		• OFF

WEEK 6

DAY 36: MONDAY	• Run for 3 miles
DAY 37: TUESDAY	• Walk or CROSS TRAIN for 30 minutes (Don't do anything that would make your muscles very sore. Would be a great active recovery day—swimming or biking)
DAY 38: WEDNESDAY	• 2 mile run
DAY 39: THURSDAY	• OFF (Or MaxT3 Core or Upper Training)
DAY 40: FRIDAY	• OFF
DAY 41: SATURDAY	• Race 5K!
DAY 42: SUNDAY	• OFF

8 WEEKS TO 10K: THE FITNESS PLAN

WEEK 1

DAY 1: MONDAY	MaxT3	• Warm-up: 10 minute walk/jog • 4 rounds of: 15 Tuck Jumps; 50 meter Sprint-Run at 90-100% effort; 20 Push-ups; Rest and Repeat (Rest 2 minutes between each set)
DAY 2: TUESDAY		• Walk 30 Minutes
DAY 3: WEDNESDAY		• Walk for 1 mile. Run for 2 minutes or walk for 5 minutes. Keep it up for 2 miles (3 miles total)
DAY 4: THURSDAY		• OFF (Or MaxT3 Core or Upper Training)
DAY 5: FRIDAY		• Walk 2 miles
DAY 6: SATURDAY		• Run for 2 minutes or walk quickly for 5 minutes for 3 miles
DAY 7: SUNDAY		• OFF

WEEK 2

DAY 8: MONDAY	*MaxT3*	• Warm-up: 10 minute walk/jog • 2 rounds of: 10 Burpees; 15 Push-ups; 25 Crunches; 10 Jump Squats; 100m Sprint-Run at 90-100% effort; Rest and Repeat (Rest 2 minutes between each set)
DAY 9: TUESDAY		• Walk 3 miles
DAY 10: WEDNESDAY		• Walk quickly for 1 mile. Run for 3 minutes or walk quickly for 5 minutes. Keep it up for 3 miles (4 miles total)
DAY 11: THURSDAY		• OFF (Or MaxT3 Core or Upper Training)
DAY 12: FRIDAY		• Run for 3 minutes or walk quickly for 5 minutes for 3 miles
DAY 13: SATURDAY		•Walk 1 mile and walk-run for 2.5 miles (Run 30 seconds, walk 1 minute). Total 3.5 miles
DAY 14: SUNDAY		• OFF

WEEK 3

DAY 15: MONDAY	*MaxT3*	• Warm-up: Jog ½ mile • 2 rounds of: 10 Squat Jumps; 15 Shin Slaps; 30 Mountain Climbers; 10 Burpees; Rest and Repeat (2 minutes rest between each set) • 3x100 meter Sprint-Runs at 90-100% effort (30 seconds rest between each set); Rest 2 minutes and Repeat 3x100 meter Run
DAY 16: TUESDAY		• Walk 3.5 miles
DAY 17: WEDNESDAY		• Walk quickly for 1 mile. Run for 10 minutes or walk quickly for 5 minutes for 3 miles (4 miles total)
DAY 18: THURSDAY		• OFF (Or MaxT3 Core or Upper Training)
DAY 19: FRIDAY		• CROSS TRAIN DAY: Walk 3.5 miles or bike/swim/elliptical/rollerblade for 30 minutes
DAY 20: SATURDAY		• Walk 1 mile and run 10 min. Walk 5 minutes for 3 miles and a total of 4 miles
DAY 21: SUNDAY		• OFF

WEEK 4

DAY 22: MONDAY	*MaxT3*	• Warm-up: Jog ½ mile • 2 rounds of (2 min. rest between each set): 10 Burpees; 25 Squat Jacks; 15 Diamond Push-ups; 20 Bodyweight Squats; Rest and Repeat • 4x100 meter Sprint-Run at 90-100% effort (60-90 second rest between every 2 rounds): Rest 2 minutes between each set
DAY 23: TUESDAY		• Walk 3.5 miles
DAY 24: WEDNESDAY		• Walk quickly for 1 mile. Run for 10 minutes or walk quickly for 5 minutes for 3 miles (4 miles total)
DAY 25: THURSDAY		• OFF (Or MaxT3 Core or Upper Training)
DAY 26: FRIDAY		• CROSS TRAIN DAY: Walk 3.5 miles or bike/swim/elliptical/rollerblade for 45 minutes
DAY 27: SATURDAY		• Run 4 miles (Run/walk if necessary)
DAY 28: SUNDAY		• OFF

WEEK 5

DAY 29: MONDAY	*MaxT3*	• Warm-up: Jog 1 mile • 100 Squat Jumps (5 minute limit); Rest 2 minutes • 3x200 meter Sprint-Run. Rest and Repeat (1-2 minutes rest between each set)
DAY 30: TUESDAY		• Walk 4 miles
DAY 31: WEDNESDAY		• Walk quickly for 1 mile. Run for 3 minutes or walk for 2 minutes for 3.5 miles (4.5 miles total)
DAY 32: THURSDAY		• OFF (Or MaxT3 Core or Upper Training)
DAY 33: FRIDAY		• CROSS TRAIN DAY: Walk 3.5 miles or bike/swim/elliptical/rollerblade for 45 minutes
DAY 34: SATURDAY		• Run for 4.5 miles
DAY 35: SUNDAY		• OFF

WEEK 6

DAY 36: MONDAY	MaxT3	• Warm-up: Jog 1 mile • 50 Tuck Jumps (4 minute limit) • 2x400 meter Sprint-Run (Rest 1 minute between each set); • Rest 2 minutes • 2x400 meter Sprint-Run (Rest 2 minutes between each set)
DAY 37: TUESDAY		• Walk 4 miles
DAY 38: WEDNESDAY		• Run for 3 miles
DAY 39: THURSDAY		• OFF (Or MaxT3 Core or Upper Training)
DAY 40: FRIDAY		• CROSS TRAIN DAY: Walk 4 miles or bike/swim/elliptical/ rollerblade for 60 minutes
DAY 41: SATURDAY		• Run 5 miles
DAY 42: SUNDAY		• OFF

WEEK 7

DAY 43: MONDAY	MaxT3	• Warm-up: Jog 1 mile • 100 Squat Jumps (5 minute limit) • 3x200 meter Sprint-Run (Rest 30 seconds between each set) • Rest 2 minutes • 3x200 meter Sprint-Run (Rest 60-90 seconds betwen each set)
DAY 44: TUESDAY		• Walk 4 miles
DAY 45: WEDNESDAY		• Run for 3 miles
DAY 46: THURSDAY		• OFF (Or MaxT3 Core or Upper Training)
DAY 47: FRIDAY		• CROSS TRAIN DAY: Walk 4 miles or bike/swim/elliptical/ rollerblade for 60 minutes
DAY 48: SATURDAY		• Run for 5.5 miles
DAY 49: SUNDAY		• OFF

WEEK 8

DAY 50: MONDAY	• Run 3 miles
DAY 51: TUESDAY	• Walk or CROSS TRAIN for 30 minutes
DAY 52: WEDNESDAY	• Run for 2 miles
DAY 53: THURSDAY	• OFF (Or MaxT3 Core or Upper Training)
DAY 54: FRIDAY	• OFF
DAY 55: SATURDAY	• RACE 10K!
DAY 56: SUNDAY	• OFF

12 WEEKS TO HALF MARATHON: THE FITNESS PLAN

WEEK 1

DAY 1: MONDAY	*MaxT3*	• Warm-up: 10 minute walk/jog • 4 rounds of:15 Tuck Jumps; 50 meter Sprint-Run at 90-100% effort; 20 Push-ups; Rest and Repeat (2 minutes rest between each set)
DAY 2: TUESDAY		• Walk 30 Minutes
DAY 3: WEDNESDAY		• Walk quickly for 1 mile. Run for 2 minutes or walk for 5 minutes. Keep it up for 2 miles (3 miles total)
DAY 4: THURSDAY		• OFF (Or MaxT3 Core or Upper Training)
DAY 5: FRIDAY		• Run for 2 minutes or walk quickly for 5 minutes for 3 miles
DAY 6: SATURDAY		• Walk 2 miles
DAY 7: SUNDAY		• OFF

WEEK 2		
DAY 8: MONDAY	*MaxT3*	• Warm-up: 10 minute walk/jog • 2 rounds of: 10 Burpees; 15 Push-ups; 25 Crunches; 10 Jump Squats; 100 meter Sprint-Run at 90-100% effort; Rest 2 minutes and Repeat (2 minutes rest between each set)
DAY 9: TUESDAY		• Walk 3 miles
DAY 10: WEDNESDAY		• Walk quickly for 1 mile. Run for 3 minutes or walk quickly for 5 minutes. Keep it up for 3 miles (4 miles total)
DAY 11: THURSDAY		• OFF (Or MaxT3 Core or Upper Training)
DAY 12: FRIDAY		• Run for 3 minutes or walk quickly for 5 minutes for 3 miles
DAY 13: SATURDAY		• Walk 1 mile and walk run for 2.5 miles (Run 30 seconds, walk 1 minute). Total 3.5 miles
DAY 14: SUNDAY		• OFF
WEEK 3		
DAY 15: MONDAY	*MaxT3*	• Warm-up: Jog ½ mile • 2 rounds of: 10 Squat Jumps; 15 Shin Slaps; 30 Mountain Climbers; 10 Burpees; Rest 2 minutes and Repeat (2 minutes rest between each set) • 3x100 meter Sprint-Run at 90-100% effort (60-90 second rest between each set): Rest 2 minutes; Repeat 3x100 meter run
DAY 16: TUESDAY		• Walk 3.5 miles
DAY 17: WEDNESDAY		• Walk quickly for 1 mile. Run for 10 minutes or walk quickly for 5 minutes for 3 miles (4 miles total)
DAY 18: THURSDAY		• OFF (Or MaxT3 Core or Upper Training)
DAY 19: FRIDAY		• CROSS TRAIN DAY: Walk 3.5 miles or bike/swim/elliptical/rollerblade for 45 minutes
DAY 20: SATURDAY		• Walk 1 mile and run 10 minutes or walk 5 minutes for 3 miles (4 miles total)
DAY 21: SUNDAY		• OFF

WEEK 4

DAY 22: MONDAY	*MaxT3*	• Warm-up: Jog ½ mile • 2 rounds of: 10 Burpees; 25 Squat Jacks; 15 Diamond Push-ups; 20 Bodyweight Squats; Rest and Repeat (2 minutes rest between each set) • 4x100 meter Sprint-Run at 90-100% effort (Rest 60-90 seconds between every 2 rounds); Rest 2 minutes between rounds
DAY 23: TUESDAY		• Walk 3.5 miles
DAY 24: WEDNESDAY		• Walk quickly for 1 mile. Run for 10 minutes or walk quickly for 5 minutes for 3 miles (4 miles total)
DAY 25: THURSDAY		• OFF (Or MaxT3 Core or Upper Training)
DAY 26: FRIDAY		• CROSS TRAIN DAY: Walk 3.5 miles or bike/swim/elliptical/rollerblade for 45 minutes
DAY 27: SATURDAY		• Run 4 miles (Run/walk if necessary)
DAY 28: SUNDAY		• OFF

WEEK 5

DAY 29: MONDAY	*MaxT3*	• Warm-up: Jog 1 mile • 100 Squat Jumps (5 minute limit); Rest 2 minutes • 3x200 meter Sprint-Run (60-90 seconds rest between each set)
DAY 30: TUESDAY		• Walk 4 miles
DAY 31: WEDNESDAY		• Walk quickly for 1 mile. Run for 3 minutes or walk for 2 minutes for 3.5 miles (4.5 miles total)
DAY 32: THURSDAY		• OFF (Or MaxT3 Core or Upper Training)
DAY 33: FRIDAY		• CROSS TRAIN DAY: Walk 4 miles or bike/swim/elliptical/rollerblade for 60 minutes
DAY 34: SATURDAY		• Run for 4.5 miles
DAY 35: SUNDAY		• OFF

WEEK 6

DAY 36: MONDAY	**MaxT3**	• Warm-up: Jog 1 mile
		• 50 Tuck Jumps (4 minutes limit)
		• 2x400 meter Sprint-Run
		  (Rest 1 minute between each set);
		• Rest 2 minutes
		• 2x400 meter Sprint-Run
		  (Rest 1-2 minutes between each set)

DAY 37: TUESDAY		• Walk 4 miles
DAY 38: WEDNESDAY		• Run for 3 miles
DAY 39: THURSDAY		• OFF (Or MaxT3 Core or Upper Training)
DAY 40: FRIDAY		• Walk 4 miles or CROSS TRAIN for 60 minutes
DAY 41: SATURDAY		• Run 5 miles
DAY 42: SUNDAY		• OFF (Or MaxT3 Core or Upper Training)

WEEK 7

DAY 43: MONDAY	**MaxT3**	• Warm-up: Jog 1 mile
		• 100 Squat Jumps (5 minute limit);
		• 3x200 meter Sprint-Run. (Rest 30 seconds
		  between each set); Rest 2 minutes
		• 3x200 meter Sprint-Run (Rest 60-90 seconds
		  betwen each set)

DAY 44: TUESDAY		• Walk 4 miles
DAY 45: WEDNESDAY		• Run for 4 miles
DAY 46: THURSDAY		• OFF (Or MaxT3 Core or Upper Training)
DAY 47: FRIDAY		• CROSS TRAIN DAY: Walk 4 miles or bike/swim/elliptical/ rollerblade for 60 minutes
DAY 48: SATURDAY		• Run for 6 miles
DAY 49: SUNDAY		• OFF

WEEK 8

DAY 50: MONDAY	*MaxT3*	• Warm-up: Jog 1 mile • 200 bodyweight squats (5 minute limit) • 3x200 meter Sprint-Run (Rest 1 minute between each set); Rest 2 minutes • 3x200 meter Sprint-Run (Rest 60-90 seconds between each set)

DAY 51: TUESDAY
• Walk 4.5 miles

DAY 52: WEDNESDAY
• Run 4 miles

DAY 53: THURSDAY
• OFF (Or MaxT3 Core or Upper Training)

DAY 54: FRIDAY
• Walk 4 miles or CROSS TRAIN for 60 minutes

DAY 55: SATURDAY
• Run 7 miles

DAY 56: SUNDAY
• OFF

WEEK 9

DAY 57: MONDAY	*MaxT3*	• Warm-up: Jog 1 mile • 3 rounds of 15 Burpees; 20 Push-ups; 30 Crunches; 20 Jump Squats; Rest 2 minutes and Repeat (2 minutes rest between each set)

DAY 58: TUESDAY
• Walk 4.5 miles

DAY 59: WEDNESDAY
• Run 4 miles

DAY 60: THURSDAY
• OFF (Or MaxT3 Core or Upper Training)

DAY 61: FRIDAY
• CROSS TRAIN DAY: Walk 4 miles or bike/swim/elliptical/rollerblade for 60 minutes

DAY 62: SATURDAY
• Run 8 miles

DAY 63: SUNDAY
• OFF

WEEK 10		
DAY 64: MONDAY	*MaxT3*	• Warm-up: Jog 1 mile • 3 rounds of 15 Burpees; 20 Push-ups; 30 Crunches; 20 Jump Squats; Rest 2 minutes and Repeat (2 minutes rest between each set)
DAY 65: TUESDAY		• Walk 5 miles
DAY 66: WEDNESDAY		• Run 4 miles
DAY 67: THURSDAY		• OFF (Or MaxT3 Core or Upper Training)
DAY 68: FRIDAY		• CROSS TRAIN DAY: Walk 4 miles or bike/swim/elliptical/ rollerblade for 60 minutes
DAY 69: SATURDAY		• Run 9 miles
DAY 70: SUNDAY		• OFF
WEEK 11		
DAY 71: MONDAY	*MaxT3*	• Warm-up: Jog 1 mile • 50 Burpees (5 minute time limit) • Sprint-Run Ladder (Rest 1-2 minutes between each run)—2x50; Rest 1 minute; 2x100; Rest 1 minute; 2x200; Rest 1 minute; 2x400
DAY 72: TUESDAY		• Walk 5 miles
DAY 73: WEDNESDAY		• Run 4 miles
DAY 74: THURSDAY		• OFF (Or MaxT3 Core or Upper Training)
DAY 75: FRIDAY		• CROSS TRAIN DAY: Walk 4 miles or bike/swim/elliptical/ rollerblade for 60 minutes
DAY 76: SATURDAY		• Run for 10 miles
DAY 77: SUNDAY		• OFF (Or MaxT3 Core or Upper Training)

DAY 78: MONDAY	• OFF
DAY 79: TUESDAY	• Run 4 miles
DAY 80: WEDNESDAY	• Walk for 30 minutes or CROSS TRAIN for 30 minutes
DAY 81: THURSDAY	• Run 2 miles
DAY 82: FRIDAY	• OFF (Or MaxT3 Core Upper Trainer)
DAY 83: SATURDAY	• OFF
DAY 84: SUNDAY	• Race Half-Marathon!

16 WEEKS TO MARATHON: THE FITNESS PLAN

This plan is 16 weeks depending on comfort level. Many marathon programs end with 18 miles for the longest run. This is a distance you will achieve by week 14 with two weeks of taper before the marathon, which will allow you to finish the race. If you're more comfortable with achieving a distance of 20 miles before the event, then you will have to start a week or two earlier. 16 weeks seems like a long time, but it's really pretty fast to get in shape for a marathon. The surest way to not finish is to get hurt. So make sure to listen to your body and go easy or rest when you need it.

WEEK 1		
DAY 1: MONDAY	*MaxT3*	• Warm-up: 10 minute walk/jog • 4 rounds of: 15 Tuck Jumps; 50m Sprint-Run at 90-100% effort; 20 Push-ups; Rest 2 minutes and Repeat (2 minutes rest between each set)
DAY 2: TUESDAY		• Walk 30 Minutes
DAY 3: WEDNESDAY		• OFF (Or MaxT3 Core or Upper Training)
DAY 4: THURSDAY		• Run or run/walk 2 miles EXAMPLE RUN/WALK: 3 minutes/2 minutes. Repeat
DAY 5: FRIDAY		• CROSS TRAIN DAY: Walk 3 miles or bike/swim/elliptical/rollerblade for 30 minutes
DAY 6: SATURDAY		• Run, jog or run/walk 3 miles
DAY 7: SUNDAY		• OFF

WEEK 2

DAY 8: MONDAY	*MaxT3*	• Warm-up: 10 minute walk/jog • 2 rounds of: 10 Burpees; 15 Push-ups; 25 Crunches; 10 Jump Squats; 100 meter Sprint-Run at 90-100% effort; Rest 2 minutes and Repeat (Rest 2 minutes between each set)
DAY 9: TUESDAY		• Walk 3 miles
DAY 10: WEDNESDAY		• OFF (Or MaxT3 Core or Upper Training)
DAY 11: THURSDAY		• Run or run/walk 2 miles
DAY 12: FRIDAY		• CROSS TRAIN DAY: Walk 3 miles or bike/swim/elliptical/ rollerblade for 30 minute
DAY 13: SATURDAY		• Run or run/walk 3 miles
DAY 14: SUNDAY		• OFF

WEEK 3

DAY 15: MONDAY	*MaxT3*	• Warm-up: Jog ½ mile • 2 rounds of (2 minutes rest between each set): 10 Squat jumps; 15 Shin Slaps; 30 Mountain Climbers; 10 Burpees; Rest 2 minutes and Repeat • 3x100 meter Sprint-Run at 90-100% effort (60-90 seconds rest between each set); Rest 2 minutes; Repeat 3x100 meter run
DAY 16: TUESDAY		• Walk 3 miles
DAY 17: WEDNESDAY		• OFF (Or MaxT3 Core or Upper Training)
DAY 18: THURSDAY		• Run or run/walk 3 miles EXAMPLE Run/Walk target: 3 minutes/1 minute
DAY 19: FRIDAY		• CROSS TRAIN DAY: Walk 3 miles or bike/swim/elliptical/ rollerblade for 30 minutes
DAY 20: SATURDAY		• Run or run/walk 4 miles
DAY 21: SUNDAY		• OFF

WEEK 4

DAY 22: MONDAY	*MaxT3*	• Warm-up: Jog ½ mile • 2 rounds of: 10 Burpees; 25 Squat Jacks; 15 Diamond Push-ups; 20 Bodyweight Squats; Rest 2 minutes and Repeat (2 minutes rest between each set) • 4x100 meter Sprint-Run at 90-100% effort (Rest 60-90 seconds between every 2 rounds)
DAY 23: TUESDAY		• Run easy or run/walk at 4 minutes/1minute for 4 miles
DAY 24: WEDNESDAY		• OFF (Or MaxT3 Core or Upper Training)
DAY 25: THURSDAY		• Run or run/walk 3 miles
DAY 26: FRIDAY		• CROSS TRAIN DAY: Walk 4 miles or bike/swim/elliptical/rollerblade for 45 minutes
DAY 27: SATURDAY		• Run or run/walk 5 miles
DAY 28: SUNDAY		• OFF

WEEK 5

DAY 29: MONDAY	*MaxT3*	• Warm-up: Jog 1 mile • 100 Squat Jumps (5 minute limit); Rest 2 minutes • 3x200 meter Sprint-Run (Rest 60-90 seconds between each set)
DAY 30: TUESDAY		• Run easy or run/walk at 4 minutes/1minute for 4 miles
DAY 31: WEDNESDAY		• OFF (Or MaxT3 Core or Upper Training)
DAY 32: THURSDAY		• Run or run/walk 4.5 miles
DAY 33: FRIDAY		• CROSS TRAIN DAY: Walk 4 miles or bike/swim/elliptical/rollerblade for 45 minutes
DAY 34: SATURDAY		• Run or run/walk 6 miles
DAY 35: SUNDAY		• OFF

WEEK 6

DAY 36: MONDAY	*MaxT3*	• Warm-up: Jog 1 mile • 50 Tuck Jumps (4 minute limit) • 2x400 meter Sprint-Run (Rest 1-2 minutes between each set); Rest 2 minutes • 2x400 meter Sprint-Run (Rest 1-2 minutes between each round)
DAY 37: TUESDAY		• Run easy or run/walk at 5 minutes/1 minute for 4 miles
DAY 38: WEDNESDAY		• OFF (Or MaxT3 Core or Upper Training)
DAY 39: THURSDAY		• Run or run/walk for 5 miles
DAY 40: FRIDAY		• CROSS TRAIN DAY: bike/swim/elliptical/ rollerblade for 60 minutes
DAY 41: SATURDAY		• Run or run/walk 7 miles
DAY 42: SUNDAY		• OFF

WEEK 7

DAY 43: MONDAY	*MaxT3*	• Warm-up: Jog 1 mile • 100 Squat Jumps (5 minute limit); • 3x200 meter Sprint-Run (Rest 60-90 seconds between each set); Rest 2 minutes • 3x200 meter Sprint-Run (Rest 60-90 seconds between each round)
DAY 44: TUESDAY		• Run easy 4 miles
DAY 45: WEDNESDAY		• OFF (Or MaxT3 Core or Upper Training)
DAY 46: THURSDAY		• Run 5 miles
DAY 47: FRIDAY		• CROSS TRAIN DAY: bike/swim/elliptical/ rollerblade for 60 minutes
DAY 48: SATURDAY		• Run 8 miles
DAY 49: SUNDAY		• OFF

WEEK 8

DAY 50: MONDAY	*MaxT3*	• Warm-up: Jog 1 mile • 200 bodyweight squats (5 minute limit) • 3x200 meter Sprint-Run (Rest 1 minute between each set); Rest 2 minutes • 3x200 meter Sprint-Run (Rest 60-90 seconds between each round)
DAY 51: TUESDAY		• Run easy 4 miles
DAY 52: WEDNESDAY		• OFF (Or MaxT3 Core or Upper Training)
DAY 53: THURSDAY		• Run 5.5 miles
DAY 54: FRIDAY		• CROSS TRAIN DAY: bike/swim/elliptical/rollerblade for 60 minutes
DAY 55: SATURDAY		• Run 9 miles
DAY 56: SUNDAY		• OFF

WEEK 9

DAY 57: MONDAY	*MaxT3*	• Warm-up: Jog 1 mile • 3 rounds of: 15 Burpees; 20 Push-ups; 30 Crunches; 20 Jump Squats; Rest 2 minutes and Repeat (2 minutes rest between each set)
DAY 58: TUESDAY		• Run easy 4 miles
DAY 59: WEDNESDAY		• OFF (Or MaxT3 Core or Upper Training)
DAY 60: THURSDAY		• Run 5.5 miles
DAY 61: FRIDAY		• CROSS TRAIN DAY: bike/swim/elliptical/rollerblade for 60 minutes
DAY 62: SATURDAY		• Run 11 miles
DAY 63: SUNDAY		• OFF

WEEK 10

DAY 64: MONDAY	**MaxT3**	• Warm-up: Jog 1 mile • 3 rounds of 15 Burpees; 20 Push-ups; 30 Crunches; 20 Jump Squats; Rest 2 minutes and Repeat (2 minutes rest between each set)
DAY 65: TUESDAY		• Run easy 4 miles
DAY 66: WEDNESDAY		• OFF (Or MaxT3 Core or Upper Training)
DAY 67: THURSDAY		• Run 6 miles
DAY 68: FRIDAY		• CROSS TRAIN DAY: bike/swim/elliptical/rollerblade for 60 minutes
DAY 69: SATURDAY		• Run 12 miles
DAY 70: SUNDAY		• OFF

WEEK 11

DAY 71: MONDAY	**MaxT3**	• Warm-up: Jog 1 mile • 50 Burpees (5 minute time limit) • Sprint-Run Ladder (Rest 1-2 minutes between each set)—2x50; Rest 1 min; 2x100; Rest 1 minute; 2x200; Rest 1 minute; 2x400
DAY 72: TUESDAY		• Run easy 4 miles
DAY 73: WEDNESDAY		• OFF (Or MaxT3 Core or Upper Training)
DAY 74: THURSDAY		• Run 6 miles
DAY 75: FRIDAY		• CROSS TRAIN DAY: bike/swim/elliptical/rollerblade for 60 minutes
DAY 76: SATURDAY		• Run 13.1 miles half-marathon race for practice or a workout
DAY 77: SUNDAY		• OFF

68

WEEK 12

DAY 78: MONDAY	**MaxT3**	• Warm-up: 10-20 minutes walk/jog • 200 bodyweight squats (5 minute limit) • 3x200 meter Sprint-Run (60-90 seconds rest between each set): 2 Minutes Recovery • 3x200 meter Sprint-Run (60-90 seconds rest between each set): 2 Minutes Recovery
DAY 79: TUESDAY		• Run easy 4 miles
DAY 80: WEDNESDAY		• OFF (Or MaxT3 Core or Upper Training)
DAY 81: THURSDAY		• Run 6 miles
DAY 82: FRIDAY		• CROSS TRAIN DAY: bike/swim/elliptical/rollerblade for 60 minutes
DAY 83: SATURDAY		• Run 15 miles
DAY 84: SUNDAY		• OFF

WEEK 13

DAY 85: MONDAY	**MaxT3**	• Warm-up: Jog 1 mile • 2 rounds of: 20 Burpees (4 minute limit); 15 Walking Lunges per leg; 15 Split Crunches per leg (2 minute rest between each set)
DAY 86: TUESDAY		• Run easy 4 miles
DAY 87: WEDNESDAY		• OFF (Or MaxT3 Core or Upper Training)
DAY 88: THURSDAY		• Run 6 miles
DAY 89: FRIDAY		• CROSS TRAIN DAY: bike/swim/elliptical/rollerblade for 60 minutes
DAY 90: SATURDAY		• Run 16 miles
DAY 91: SUNDAY		• OFF

WEEK 14

DAY 92: MONDAY	*MaxT3*	• Warm-up: Jog mile • 2 rounds of: 20 Burpees; 20 Push-ups; 50 meter Sprint; 30 Crunches, 20 Jump Squats; 50 meter Sprint; Rest 2 minutes and Repeat (2 minutes rest between each set)
DAY 93: TUESDAY	• Run easy 4 miles	
DAY 94: WEDNESDAY	• OFF (Or MaxT3 Core or Upper Training)	
DAY 95: THURSDAY	• Run 6 miles	
DAY 96: FRIDAY	• CROSS TRAIN DAY: bike/swim/elliptical/rollerblade for 60 minutes	
DAY 97: SATURDAY	• Run 18 miles	
DAY 98: SUNDAY	• OFF	

WEEK 15

DAY 99: MONDAY	• Run an easy 4 miles
DAY 100: TUESDAY	• OFF (Or MaxT3 Core or Upper Training)
DAY 101: WEDNESDAY	• Run 3 miles
DAY 102: THURSDAY	• OFF
DAY 103: FRIDAY	• CROSS TRAIN DAY: bike/swim/elliptical/rollerblade for 60 minutes
DAY 104: SATURDAY	• Run 8 miles
DAY 105: SUNDAY	• OFF

WEEK 16

DAY 106: MONDAY	• Run 5 miles
DAY 107: TUESDAY	• OFF
DAY 108: WEDNESDAY	• Run 3 miles
DAY 109: THURSDAY	• Walk 2 miles
DAY 110: FRIDAY	• OFF
DAY 111: SATURDAY	• MARATHON RACE DAY!!!!!
DAY 112: SUNDAY	• OFF

30-Day Meal Plan: The Recipes and Beyond

Breakfast and Smoothies

Breakfast Recipe: Berry Breakfast Smoothie
- Servings: 1 (serving size: 8 ounce smoothie)
- Total time (prep to finish): 5 minutes

Ingredients
- 1 cup fresh berries of choice (strawberries, blackberries, raspberries, etc., or a combination of mixed berries)
- ½ cup coconut milk
- ½ cup crushed ice and/or water (as needed for desired thickness)
- 1 scoop Vanilla Perfect Protein powder
- ½ cup flax seeds and/or chia seeds

Directions
1. In a blender, combine the contents and process until smooth, adding more crushed ice or water as needed to achieve desired thickness.
2. Pour the smoothie into a tall glass and drink immediately to receive full nutritional value—the nutrients will begin to dissipate the longer the smoothie is exposed to the air.

Nutritional Data
- Calories: 278
- Total Fat: 20 (saturated fat: 10; polyunsaturated fat: 4.3; monounsaturated fat: 1.1)
- Carbohydrates: 17
- Fiber: 7
- Protein: 28

Breakfast Recipe: Chocolate-Covered Strawberry Smoothie
- Servings: 1 (serving size: 8 ounce smoothie)
- Total time (prep to finish): 5 minutes

Ingredients
- ½ cup coconut milk
- 1-2 cups crushed ice, depending on desired thickness/consistency
- ½ avocado, peeled, stone removed and discarded; flesh chopped
- ½ cup fresh strawberries, hulled and quartered
- 2 tablespoons unsweetened cocoa powder
- 1 scoop Chocolate Perfect Protein powder

Directions

1. In a blender, combine the contents and process until smooth, adding more crushed ice or water as needed to achieve desired thickness.
2. Pour the smoothie into a tall glass and drink immediately to receive full nutritional value—the nutrients will begin to dissipate the longer the smoothie is exposed to the air.

Nutritional Data

- Calories: 489
- Total Fat: 41
- Carbohydrates: 26
- Fiber: 16
- Protein: 29

....

Breakfast Recipe: Nutrition Knock-Out Green Smoothie

- Servings: 1 (serving size: 8 ounce green smoothie)
- Total time (prep to finish): 5 minutes

Ingredients

- 1 cup filtered water
- 1 cup fresh strawberries, hulled and quartered
- 2 cups romaine lettuce, chopped
- 2 tablespoons lemongrass, chopped
- ½ teaspoon ground flaxseed
- 1 scoop Vanilla Perfect Protein powder
- 4-6 ice cubes, or as needed

Directions

1. In a blender, combine the water, strawberries, romaine lettuce, lemongrass, and the ice cubes.
2. Process just until smooth and then add in the ground flaxseed and protein powder; process again for 5-10 seconds or until well incorporated.
3. Add additional ice, if needed until desired consistency is achieved.
4. Pour the green smoothie into tall glass and drink immediately to receive full nutritional value—the nutrients will begin to dissipate the longer the smoothie is exposed to the air.

Nutritional Data

- Calories: 162
- Total Fat: 5
- Carbohydrates: 15
- Fiber: 7
- Protein: 22

Breakfast Recipe: Cherry Vanilla Green Smoothie
- Servings: 1 (serving size: 8 ounce green smoothie)
- Total time (prep to finish): 5 minutes

Ingredients
- ½ cup coconut milk
- 1 cup organic frozen cherries, pitted
- 1 cup Spirulina (optional)
- 1 cup raw spinach
- 1 scoop Vanilla Perfect Protein Powder
- ½ cup So Delicious (or preferred brand) dairy-free coconut milk-based Greek yogurt, vanilla flavored
- 5-6 ice cubes (optional)

Directions
1. Place the coconut milk, cherries, Spirulina, yogurt, and the ice (optional) into the blender. Cover and blend until smooth, stopping frequently to push down any ingredients that may have stuck to the blender walls.
2. Pour into a tall glass and drink immediately to receive full nutritional value.

Nutritional Data
- Calories: 382
- Total Fat: 29
- Carbohydrates: 19
- Fiber: 1
- Protein: 39

....

Breakfast Recipe: Strawberries & Spinach Green Smoothie
This is a great Cost-Conscious Meal. A pint of strawberries and one bunch of baby spinach costs less than $5 and can be divided and spread out to make smoothies, such as this one; as well as simple salads, sandwiches/wraps, and many more meals.
- Servings: 1 (serving size: 8 ounce green smoothie)
- Total Time (prep to finish): 5 minutes

Ingredients
- 1 cup baby spinach
- 1 cup fresh strawberries, hulled and quartered
- 1 scoop Vanilla Perfect Protein Powder
- ½ avocado, peeled
- ½-1 cup coconut water (or filtered water)
- 1 cup crushed ice, as needed to achieve desired thickness

Directions

1. Place ingredients in blender in order listed.
2. Cover and blend until smooth, stopping frequently to push down any ingredients that may have stuck to the blender walls.
3. Pour into a tall glass and drink immediately to receive full nutritional value.

Nutritional Data

- Calories: 304
- Total Fat: 30
- Carbohydrates: 16
- Fiber: 13
- Protein: 33

....

Breakfast Recipe: Spinach and Egg Omelet

- Servings: 2 one-ounce omelets
- Total time (prep to finish): 20 minutes

Ingredients

- 2 large pasture-raised eggs
- 1 cup baby spinach, chopped or torn
- Sea salt, to taste
- Fresh ground black pepper, to taste
- 1 teaspoon coconut oil

Directions

1. Place a 10-inch non-stick skillet over medium-low heat. Melt the coconut oil in the skillet.
2. In a small bowl, whisk together the eggs, salt, and black pepper. Pour the beaten eggs into the skillet, and swirl the pan around to help spread the eggs out.
3. When the omelet is nearly set, but still has a little raw egg left on the surface, sprinkle on the torn spinach and then use a spatula to carefully peel up the edges of the eggs and fold in half. Continue cooking until set. Then transfer to plate and enjoy!

Nutritional Data

- Calories: 207
- Total Fat: 13
- Carbohydrates: 2
- Fiber: 0
- Protein: 12

....

Breakfast Recipe: 2 Eggs and an Avocado

Here is another great Cost-Conscious Meal. A dozen eggs can make for easy, cost-effective meals that can be very versatile.

- Servings: 1 (serving size: 2 eggs and ½ avocado)
- Total time (prep to finish): 10 minutes

Ingredients

- 2 large pasture-raised eggs, cooked to order
- ½ ripe avocado, sliced

Directions

1. In a 10-inch nonstick skillet or frying pan, cook eggs according to preference.
2. Slice the avocado and serve alongside the eggs.

Nutritional Data

- Calories: 271
- Total Fat: 24
- Carbohydrates: 10
- Fiber: 7
- Protein: 7

....

Breakfast Recipe: Scrambled Eggs with Apple

- Servings: 1 (serving size: 2 eggs, ½ apple)
- Total time (prep to finish): 10 minutes

Ingredients

- 2 large pasture-raised eggs
- ½ Granny Smith apple, cored and cut into wedges
- Sea salt (to taste)
- Fresh ground black pepper (to taste)

Directions

1. Do not cut the apple until ready to serve to keep the wedges fresh.
2. Place the eggs into a shallow bowl with the salt and black pepper. Whisk lightly just until beaten, then pour the beaten egg into the skillet and scramble for about 3-5 minutes, or until desired doneness is achieved.
3. Core and wedge the apple and arrange ½ of the apple wedges next to the eggs. Sprinkle with additional sea salt and black pepper, to taste, and then serve and enjoy.

Nutritional Data

- Calories: 168
- Total Fat: 9

- Carbohydrates: 17
- Fiber: 3
- Protein: 5

Breakfast Recipe: Fried Eggs and Cherry Tomatoes

- Servings: 1 (serving size: 2 eggs; 1 cup cherry tomatoes)
- Total time (prep to finish): 10 minutes

Ingredients

- ½ tablespoon coconut oil
- Sea salt (to taste)
- Fresh ground black pepper (to taste)
- 2 large pasture-raised eggs
- 1 cup cherry tomatoes

Directions

1. Heat the ½ tablespoon coconut oil in a skillet, and let melt over medium heat. Add the eggs and space them about 1 inch apart. S prinkle lightly, to season, with sea salt and black pepper. Cook until desired doneness is achieved.
2. Place the fried eggs on a serving plate, and serve alongside 1 cup cherry tomatoes.

Nutritional Data

- Calories: 205
- Total Fat: 15
- Carbohydrates: 8
- Fiber: 2
- Protein: 13

Breakfast Recipe: "Kitchen Sink" Yogurt

Here's another Cost-Conscious Meal—simple, inexpensive breakfast of yogurt and fresh berries at less than $2.00 per serving!

- Servings: 1 (serving size: 1 cup yogurt; ½ cup fresh berries)
- Total Time (prep to finish): 5 minutes

Ingredients

- 1 cup organic whole (or goat's milk) plain yogurt
- 1-2 teaspoons shaved unsweetened raw chocolate
- ⅛ teaspoon Stevia, to taste
- ¼ cup ground flax seed and/or chia seeds
- 1-2 tablespoons shredded coconut (optional)
- 1 teaspoon almond or peanut butter

- ½ cup fresh strawberries, raspberries, blueberries, or a combination of mixed berries

Directions

1. Combine all ingredients except for the fresh berries into a bowl. Stir to mix well
2. Fold in ½ of the berries, and stir gently. Then sprinkle the top of the yogurt with the remaining berries.
3. Enjoy!

Nutritional Data

- Calories: 325
- Total Fat: 17
- Carbohydrates: 27
- Fiber: 11
- Protein: 11

Breakfast Recipe: Vegetable and Egg Breakfast Scramble

- Servings: 1 (serving size: 2 scrambled eggs with veggies)
- Total Time (prep to finish): 15 minutes

Ingredients

- 2 large pasture-raised eggs
- ¼ cup white onion, chopped
- ½ cup raw spinach, chopped fine (optional)
- Sea salt (to taste)
- White pepper (to taste)

Directions

1. In a small mixing bowl, add the eggs and beat lightly; whisk in the sea salt and white pepper.
2. Place a medium-sized nonstick skillet over medium-low heat. Pour the beaten eggs into the skillet and cook, stirring often, for 3-5 minutes or until the eggs begin to scramble. When the eggs are nearly done, toss in the veggies, and gently stir to incorporate. Continue cooking until eggs are set, vegetables are heated through, and the spinach is slightly wilted.
3. Transfer the scrambled eggs to a serving dish, sprinkle on a little more sea salt and white pepper, if desired, to taste, and then serve immediately.

Nutritional Data

- Calories: 136
- Total Fat: 8
- Carbohydrates: 5

- Fiber: 1
- Protein: 13

Breakfast Recipe: 2 Eggs and Fresh Berries
- Servings: 1 (serving size: 2 eggs; 1 cup fresh berries)
- Total Time (prep to finish): 10 minutes

Ingredients
- 2 large pasture-raised eggs, cooked as desired
- 1 cup fresh berries

Directions
1. In a 10-inch nonstick skillet or frying pan, cook eggs according to preference.
2. Rinse 1 cup of fresh berries and serve alongside the eggs.

Nutritional Data
- Calories: 200
- Total Fat: 9
- Carbohydrates: 13
- Fiber: 5
- Protein: 13

Breakfast Recipe: Eggnog Smoothie
- Servings: 1 (serving size: 8 ounces)
- Total Time (prep to finish): 5 minutes

Ingredients
- 1 scoop Vanilla Perfect Protein Powder
- ½ can coconut milk (full-fat)
- ½ avocado
- 1-2 cups ice (for desired thickness and consistency)
- 1 teaspoon vanilla extract
- 2 teaspoons ground nutmeg and cinnamon
- Stevia (to taste)

Directions
1. Add all ingredients into the blender. Blend on high until creamy and frothy.
2. Serve immediately.

Nutritional Data
- Calories: 497
- Total Fat: 43
- Carbohydrates: 17

- Fiber: 13
- Protein: 29

....

Breakfast Recipe: Grain-less Granola
- Servings: 2 (serving size: ½ cup)
- Total Time (prep to finish): 5 minutes

Ingredients
- ¼ cup whole organic flax seeds
- ¼ cup raw organic almonds
- ¼ cup dry, unsweetened coconut
- 2 teaspoons dried mint leaves or 2 mint tea bags
- ½ cup chilled coconut milk

Directions
1. In blender or food processor, pour flax seeds, almonds, and dry coconut through opening in top of cover. Replace removable cap, and continue processing until ingredients are reduced to a chunky, grain-like consistency, about 1 minute. Stop motor, and scrape down to loosen mixture in bottom of blender or bowl, if necessary.
2. Add loose, dry mint leaves, or open 2 mint tea bags, and dump contents. Process a few more bursts until blended.
3. Can be enjoyed cold, or let stand a few minutes, and warm slightly on stovetop for a "hot" cereal experience. Flax seeds will thicken mixture as it sits.

Nutritional Data
- Calories: 265
- Total Fat: 20 (6 grams monounsaturated; 10 grams saturated; 5 grams polyunsaturated)
- Carbohydrates: 12
- Fiber: 8
- Protein: 9

....

Breakfast Recipe: Blueberry Muffins
- Servings: 10 (serving size: 1 muffin)
- Total Time (prep to finish): 35-40 minutes

Ingredients
- 3 pasture-raised eggs
- ½ cup whole milk Greek yogurt
- ⅓ cup grapeseed oil
- ½ cup Xylitol

- 1 tablespoon vanilla extract
- ½ cup coconut flour
- ¼ teaspoon sea salt
- ¼ teaspoon baking soda
- ½-1 cup fresh or frozen blueberries

Directions

1. Preheat oven to 350°F; line muffin tins.
2. In a food processor combine eggs, yogurt, oil, vanilla and Xylitol. Pulse until mixed.
3. Pulse in coconut flour, salt, and baking soda. Add blueberries, and pulse two or three times to break up slightly.
4. Fill lined muffin tins. Bake for 20-25 minutes until tops are slightly browned. Makes 10 muffins.

Nutritional Data (per muffin)

- Calories: 145
- Total Fat: 10 (5 grams monounsaturated; 3 grams saturated; 2 grams polyunsaturated)
- Carbohydrates: 9
- Fiber: 4
- Protein: 5

Breakfast Recipe: Brownie Cereal

Ingredients

- 1-½ cups unsweetened shredded coconut
- ⅓ cup unsweetened coconut milk
- ¼ cup unsweetened cocoa powder
- ½ teaspoon liquid or powder Stevia to taste
- ½ teaspoon vanilla extract

Directions

1. Preheat oven to 350°F.
2. Blend the coconut milk and cocoa powder in a stainless steel pot at medium heat.
3. Add in the Stevia, vanilla extract and shredded coconut until it's all blended in. Remove from heat.
4. Spread mixture into a thin layer on a parchment on a baking sheet.
5. Bake at 350°F for 25-30 minutes dependent on how crunchy you like it.
6. Stir the granola about 15 minutes, and make sure it doesn't burn. Store in airtight container.

Breakfast Recipe: Coconut Pancakes with Blueberries

- Servings: 1 (serving size: 2 pancakes)
- Total Time (prep to finish): 10 minutes

Ingredients

- 1 pasture-raised egg
- ¼ cup coconut milk
- ¼ cup water
- ½ teaspoon baking soda
- ¼ cup coconut flour
- ¼ cup fresh blueberries
- 1 tablespoon unsweetened shredded coconut (optional)
- ½ tablespoon coconut oil

Directions

1. In a large mixing bowl, combine the egg, coconut milk, water, baking soda, and coconut flour. Whisk contents together just until blended and a good pancake batter is formed. Be careful to not over mix.
2. Fold in the blueberries and coconut (if using) until incorporated. Let batter sit for a couple minutes while you prepare the griddle.
3. Heat a griddle with coconut oil over medium heat. When the oil has melted, pour ¼ cup batter onto the griddle. Fit as many pancakes on the griddle as possible without them touching and still allowing enough room to be able to flip each pancake with a spatula.
4. Let the pancakes cook for 3-4 minutes, then when bubbles appear along the surface, flip the pancakes and cook the other side for 2-3 minutes or until golden brown.
5. Serve and enjoy.

Nutritional Data (per 2 pancakes)

- Calories: 364
- Total Fat: 27
- Carbohydrates: 14
- Fiber: 2
- Sugars: 8
- Protein: 7

Breakfast Recipe: Waffles with Mixed Berries

- Servings: 1 (serving size: 2 waffles)
- Total time (prep to finish): 10 minutes

Ingredients

- ¼ cup blanched almond flour
- ⅛ cup tapioca starch (or arrowroot powder, if preferred)
- ⅛ tablespoon plus ⅛ teaspoon baking powder
- ½ tablespoon coconut palm sugar
- ⅛ teaspoon sea salt, or to taste
- 1 pasture-raised egg
- ½ tablespoon coconut oil, melted
- ⅛ cup coconut milk
- ¼ teaspoon fresh-squeezed lemon juice
- ¼ teaspoon vanilla extract
- ½ tablespoon almond butter (or preferred toppings)
- ¼ cup fresh mixed berries of choice (blueberries, strawberries, raspberries, blackberries, etc.)

Directions

1. Preheat your waffle iron.
2. In a mixing bowl, combine all of the ingredients in the order listed (except for the almond butter and mixed berries) and mix until just barely combined, a few remaining lumps are fine. Let the waffle batter set at room temperature for 5 minutes.
3. Using a ladle, scoop approximately ¼ cup of the batter (or the amount indicated by the waffle iron's manufacturer) onto your hot waffle iron. Cook the waffles according to the manufacturer directions for your particular waffle iron or for 4-6 minutes or until preferred doneness/ crispiness is reached.
4. Place the 2 waffles on a serving plate, add on the almond butter or desired toppings and then top the waffles with the fresh mixed berries. Note: For super-quick breakfasts, make a large batch of waffles and freeze them. Then, just pull them out of the freezer and place in the toaster or toaster oven to reheat.

Nutritional Data

- Calories: 225
- Total Fat: 16
- Carbohydrates: 21
- Fiber: 2
- Sugars: 8
- Protein: 10

Lunch

Lunch Recipe: Grilled Chicken Chopped Salad

- Servings: 1 (serving size: 2 cups salad with 4-6 ounces grilled chicken breasts)
- Total time (prep to finish): 20 minutes

Ingredients

- One 4-6 ounce free-range boneless, skinless chicken breast
- Pinch of sea salt
- Pinch of fresh ground black pepper
- 1-2 tablespoons extra virgin olive oil
- 2 cups mixed greens of choice, chopped
- ½ cup radishes, trimmed, chopped
- ¼ cup celery, chopped
- 1 chopped green onion (both white and green parts)
- 1 chopped red onion
- 2 tablespoons olive oil or preferred vegan dressing

Directions

1. Preheat grill to medium-high heat.
2. Cut any excess/visible fat from the chicken breasts, and rinse the chicken breasts in cool running water; pat dry with paper towels. Sprinkle with sea salt, black pepper, and drizzle on the olive oil. Grill chicken for 5-6 minutes per side or until cooked through and juices run clear. Transfer to a cutting board; let rest 3-5 minutes; chop.
3. While the chicken is grilling, prepare the other ingredients as directed. In a large salad bowl, combine the chopped grilled chicken, chopped greens, and chopped veggies. Toss/stir to combine.
4. Drizzle on olive oil or preferred vegan dressing. Toss to coat. Transfer salad to a serving dish, serve, and enjoy!

Nutritional Data

- Calories: 392
- Total Fat: 18
- Carbohydrates: 17
- Fiber: 5
- Protein: 37

Lunch Recipe: Vegetable Kabobs with Pesto

- To be served with pre-cooked char-grilled chicken.
- Servings: 1-2 (serving size: 3 vegetable kabobs with ½ cup pesto)
- Total time (prep to finish): 30 minutes

Ingredients
- ½ eggplant, cut into chunks
- ½-1 zucchini, cut into chunks
- 1 bell pepper, cut into chunks
- 1 pint cherry tomatoes
- 1 red onion, cut into quarters
- ½-1 cup preferred pesto, divided
- 3-6 bamboo skewers, presoaked in water for 20 minutes

Directions
1. Place the bamboo skewers in cool water to soak for 20 minutes.
2. Prepare vegetables as directed.
3. Preheat the grill to medium-high heat.
4. Place the veggies in a large bowl. Pour ½ cup of the pesto into the bowl over the vegetables, and toss until the vegetables are completely coated.
5. Skewer the vegetables in desired order onto each bamboo skewer, and grill for 5-7 minutes, turning as needed, until the veggies are lightly charred and fork tender.
6. Place 3 veggie kabobs on a serving dish alongside the remaining ½ cup pesto, to serve.
7. Freeze any remaining kabobs to be used as desired.

Nutritional Data
- Calories: 331
- Total Fat: 16
- Carbohydrates: 38
- Fiber: 18
- Protein: 22

....

Lunch Recipe: Vegetable Ratatouille
- Servings: 4 (serving size: 1½ to 2 cups)
- Total time (prep to finish): 10 minutes

Ingredients
- 3 tablespoons coconut oil
- 1 onion, thinly sliced
- 3 red bell peppers, thinly sliced
- 3 cloves garlic, crushed
- 1 eggplant, chopped
- 3 zucchini, sliced diagonally
- 1½ tablespoons red wine vinegar
- 2-3 large tomatoes, chopped
- ¾ cup cold water

- Sea salt (to taste)
- Fresh ground black pepper (to taste)

Directions

1. Place the coconut oil in a Dutch oven or a large, heavy-bottomed sauce-pan. Let the oil heat up over medium-high heat. Add in the red bell pepper, garlic, and onion. Sauté for 2 minutes or until softened.
2. While the pepper/onion is sautéing, chop up the eggplant, and slice the zucchini, diagonally, into rounds. Add the eggplant and zucchini to the pepper/onion, and stir to combine. Let sauté for 2 more minutes or just until just softened.
3. Next, add in the vinegar and chopped tomato. Cook for 30 seconds, stirring constantly, until the vinegar has evaporated. Add in ¼ cup cold water, season with salt and black pepper and bring to a simmer. Allow the ratatouille to simmer, covered, for 4 minutes or until the sauce has thickened and the vegetables are fork-tender.
4. Place 2 cups ratatouille on each serving plate and enjoy!

Nutritional Data

- Calories: 194
- Total Fat: 11
- Carbohydrates: 22
- Fiber: 10
- Protein: 5

Lunch Recipe: Turkey Cheese Burger on Bibb Lettuce

- Servings: 4 (serving size: 1 turkey burger)
- Total time (prep to finish): 15 minutes

Ingredients

- 1-lb. organic ground turkey
- Pinch of sea salt (to taste)
- Pinch of fresh ground black pepper (to taste)
- Pinch of crushed red pepper flakes (to taste)
- 4 slices raw cheese of choice
- 1-2 large Bibb lettuce leaves per burger patty
- 1 avocado, peeled, stone removed/discarded and the flesh sliced (optional)

Directions

1. Form the turkey into 4 patties. Sprinkle with the sea salt, black pepper, and crushed red pepper flakes.
2. Place a large skillet over medium heat. Add in the turkey burger patties and cook for 5-7 minutes per side or until the sides are nicely browned

and the patties are cooked through.

3. Place a slice of raw cheese over each patty and cook for 1-2 minutes more or just until the cheese begins to melt.

4. Lay 2 slices of Bibb lettuce on a serving plate. Transfer the turkey burger on top of the lettuce and top with the sliced avocado, if using. Serve and enjoy!

Nutritional Data
- Calories: 434
- Total Fat: 31
- Carbohydrates: 5
- Fiber: 4
- Protein: 39

....

Lunch Recipe:
Cucumber and Apple Salad with Char-grilled Chicken
- Servings: 1 (serving size: 2 cups salad with 4-6 ounces chicken)
- Total time (prep to finish): 10 minutes

Ingredients
- Leftover (4-6 ounces) char-grilled chicken (from previous night's dinner), reheated and sliced into cubes
- ½ medium Granny Smith apple, chopped
- ½ cup cucumber, chopped
- 2 cups green leaf lettuce, chopped
- 2 tablespoons extra-virgin olive oil
- 2 tablespoons balsamic vinegar

Directions
1. Prepare ingredients as directed.

2. Reheat the chicken in either the microwave or in a skillet for 2-4 minutes (depending on method) or until heated through. Transfer to a cutting board, and cut the reheated char-grilled chicken into cubes.

3. In a salad bowl, combine the chicken, green leaf lettuce, chopped apple, and chopped cucumber. Toss/stir to mix well.

4. Drizzle on the oil and vinegar. Toss to mix well.

5. Transfer to a serving plate and enjoy!

Nutritional Data
- Calories: 457
- Total Fat: 31
- Carbohydrates: 18
- Fiber: 12
- Protein: 27

Lunch Recipe:
Char-grilled Chicken, Blackberry and Baby Arugula Salad

With this Cost-Conscious Meal, a pint of mixed berries and a bag of mixed greens costs less than $5 and can be divided and spread out to make smoothies, simple salads, sandwiches, wraps, and more!

- Servings: 2 (serving size: 2 cups salad)
- Total time (prep to finish): 10 minutes

Ingredients

- Leftover (4-6 ounces) char-grilled chicken from previous night's dinner, reheated and sliced into cubes
- ½ cup fresh blackberries
- 2 cups baby arugula, chopped
- 2 tablespoons lemon juice per salad
- 2 tablespoons balsamic vinegar per salad

Directions

1. Prepare ingredients as directed.
2. Reheat the chicken in either the microwave or in a skillet for 2-4 minutes (depending on method) or until heated through. Transfer to a cutting board, and cut the reheated char-grilled chicken into cubes.
3. In a salad bowl, combine baby arugula and fresh blackberries.
4. Drizzle on the lemon juice and vinegar and toss to blend salad contents.
5. Transfer to a serving dish and enjoy.
6. Store the remaining baby arugula and blackberries in sealable stay-fresh containers, and place in the refrigerator to be used as directed throughout the 30-day meal plan. When ready to serve, just remove from refrigerator, toss/stir to revive the salad, add on the lemon juice and vinegar, then enjoy!

Nutritional Data

- Calories: 212
- Total Fat: 4
- Carbohydrates: 15
- Fiber: 8
- Protein: 29

Lunch Recipe: Grilled Salmon Salad with Blueberries and Mint
- Servings: 1 (Serving Size: 2 cups salad; 4-6 ounces grilled salmon)
- Total time (prep to finish): 20 minutes

Ingredients
- 4-6 ounces leftover wild caught grilled salmon from previous night's dinner (reheated, if desired) and broken into bite-size pieces
- 2 cups baby spinach, chopped or torn
- ½ cup fresh blueberries
- 1-2 tablespoons fresh mint, torn
- Juice from 1 lemon
- 2 tablespoons extra virgin olive oil

Directions
1. Reheat the salmon, if desired, or serve it chilled. Break the salmon into bite-size pieces.
2. In a salad bowl, combine the baby spinach, blueberries, and fresh mint. Toss to mix.
3. Drizzle on the olive oil and toss again to blend salad contents.
4. Transfer salad to a serving dish, arrange the pieces of grilled salmon over the salad, and then drizzle the lemon juice over the salmon and salad. Enjoy!

Nutritional Data
- Calories: 408
- Total Fat: 30
- Carbohydrates: 13
- Fiber: 4
- Protein: 26

Lunch Recipe: Kale, Arugula, and Spiced Steak Salad
- Servings: 1 (serving size: 2 cups salad; 4-6 ounces steak; ⅛ to ¼ cup dressing)
- Total time (prep to finish): 20 minutes

Ingredients
- 4-6 ounces Spiced Steak (leftover from previous night's dinner), reheated and sliced into thin strips.
- ½ cup baby kale, stems removed, chopped and divided
- 1½ cups baby arugula, chopped
- 3 cherry tomatoes, sliced
- 1-2 tablespoons extra-virgin olive oil
- 1-2 tablespoons balsamic vinegar per salad

Directions

1. Wash and prepare the salad ingredients as directed.
2. Reheat the steak strips either in the microwave or in a skillet for 2-4 minutes (depending on method) or until heated through. Transfer to a cutting board, and slice the steak into thin strips.
3. In a salad bowl, toss together the chopped baby kale, baby arugula, and sliced cherry tomatoes. Drizzle the olive oil and balsamic vinegar over the salad contents, and sprinkle a pinch of sea salt and black pepper, if desired. Then toss to mix.
4. Transfer salad to a serving dish; arrange the steak strips over the salad, then serve and enjoy.

Nutritional Data

- Calories: 363
- Total Fat: 18
- Carbohydrates: 24
- Fiber: 6
- Protein: 31

Lunch Recipe:

Spinach and Toasted Walnut Salad with Baked Chicken

- Servings: 1 (serving size: 2 cups salad; 4-6 ounces baked chicken breast)
- Total time (prep to finish): 10 minutes

Ingredients

- 4-6 ounces leftover baked chicken breast, reheated
- 2 cups baby spinach
- ⅛ cup walnuts, chopped coarsely
- 1 tablespoon extra-virgin olive oil
- 1 tablespoon balsamic vinegar
- ⅛ clove garlic, crushed
- ⅛ teaspoon ground cinnamon (optional)

Directions

1. Reheat the leftover baked chicken breast in the oven or microwave. Time varies depending on method: 1½ to 3 minutes in microwave on high power (100%), or 10 to 15 minutes in the oven at 350°F, or until heated throughout.
2. Meanwhile, place a small skillet over medium-low heat. Drop in the chopped walnuts and stir constantly for 3-5 minutes or until the walnuts are nicely (lightly) toasted.
3. Next, combine the olive oil, vinegar, crushed garlic, and cinnamon (if using) in a small bowl and whisk to blend well.

4. Place the spinach and toasted walnuts in a salad bowl and toss/stir to mix. Drizzle the dressing over the surface of the salad, and toss to incorporate.

5. Transfer the salad to a serving dish, serve alongside the char-grilled chicken breast and enjoy!

Nutritional Data
- Calories: 582
- Total Fat: 46
- Carbohydrates: 7
- Fiber: 3
- Protein: 36

....

Lunch Recipe:
Mixed Greens and Tilapia Salad with Macadamia Nuts

Here's another Cost-Conscious Meal. Combining a bag of mixed greens with leftover meat or fish can make an inexpensive and filling salad that you can enjoy at home, at work, or on the go!

- Servings: 1 (serving size: 2 cups salad with 4-6 ounces tilapia)
- Total time (prep to finish): 10 minutes

Ingredients
- Leftover (4-6 ounces) broiled tilapia from previous night's dinner, reheated and broken into bite-size pieces.
- 2 cups mixed greens of choice, chopped
- 1-2 tablespoons macadamia nuts, chopped
- 2 tablespoons extra virgin olive oil, for dressing

Directions
1. Reheat the tilapia in the microwave for 1-2 minutes or until heated through. Transfer to a cutting board, and break the fillet into smaller, bite-size pieces.

2. In a salad bowl, place the mixed greens. Arrange the pieces of tilapia over the greens.

3. Sprinkle the salad with the chopped macadamia nuts to garnish.

4. Finally, drizzle the salad with the olive oil as a dressing and enjoy!

Nutritional Data
- Calories: 407
- Total Fat: 35
- Carbohydrates: 3
- Fiber: 2
- Protein: 24

Lunch Recipe: Char-grilled Chicken Salad with White Beets

Cost-Conscious Meal: Adding leftover grilled chicken from dinner to liven up a simple salad makes for a fulfilling and super inexpensive lunch!

- Servings: 1 (serving size: 4-6 ounces chicken; 2 cups salad)
- Total time (prep to finish): 15 minutes

Ingredients

- 4-6 ounces leftover char-grilled chicken breast, reheated and cut into strips
- 2 cups romaine lettuce, chopped
- 3 cherry tomatoes, halved
- 1 to 2 white beets, sliced
- 2 tablespoons balsamic vinegar
- 2 tablespoons extra virgin olive oil (optional)

Directions

1. Prepare ingredients as directed.
2. Reheat the chicken in either the microwave or in a skillet for 2 to 4 minutes (depending on method) or until heated through. Transfer to a cutting board, and cut the reheated char-grilled chicken into thin strips.
3. Meanwhile, in a large salad bowl, combine the romaine lettuce, white beets, and halved cherry tomatoes. Toss to mix well. Drizzle the balsamic vinegar (and olive oil, if using) over the salad contents. Toss well to mix.
4. Transfer the salad to a serving dish and arrange 6 ounces of the char-grilled chicken breast strips over the salad and serve.
5. Place the remaining salad/chicken in a stay-fresh container, and store in the refrigerator, to be used as directed during the 30-day meal plan.

Nutritional Data

- Calories: 468
- Total Fat: 32
- Carbohydrates: 18
- Fiber: 5
- Protein: 29

Lunch Recipe:
Strawberry, Romaine, and Avocado Salad with Spiced Steak Strips

- Servings: 1 (serving size: 2 cups salad; 4-6 ounces steak)
- Total time (prep to finish): 10 minutes

Ingredients

- Leftover (4-6 ounces) Spiced Steak from previous night's dinner, re-heated and sliced into thin strips
- 1 cup fresh strawberries, hulled and halved
- 2 cups romaine lettuce, chopped
- ¼-½ ripe avocado, peeled with stone removed; sliced
- 1 tablespoon toasted walnuts, chopped coarsely
- 1 tablespoon balsamic vinegar
- 1 tablespoon extra virgin olive oil

Directions

1. Wash and prepare the salad ingredients as directed.
2. Reheat the steak strips either in the microwave or in a skillet for 2 to 4 minutes (depending on method) or until heated through.
3. In a large salad bowl, combine the halved berries, chopped romaine, and toasted walnuts. Toss to mix.
4. Transfer 2 cups of the salad to a serving dish.
5. Drizzle on the oil and vinegar; toss to mix. Arrange the reheated steak strips and desired amount of sliced avocado over the salad, then serve and enjoy!

Nutritional Data

- Calories: 692
- Total Fat: 46
- Carbohydrates: 27
- Fiber: 13
- Protein: 13

Lunch Recipe:
Italian Sautéed Fennel & Radicchio Salad with Grilled Chicken

- Servings: 1 (serving size: 4-6 ounces grilled chicken strips; 1½ cups salad)
- Total time (prep to finish): 20 minutes

Ingredients

- 4-6 ounces fully-cooked grilled chicken breast strips, heated throughout
- 3-5 tablespoons red wine vinegar

- 2 small garlic cloves, finely chopped
- 1 large fennel bulb, sliced
- ½ tablespoon coconut oil
- 1-2 small heads of radicchio, sliced or chopped to yield 2 cups
- 1½ teaspoons sea salt, divided, plus more to taste, if needed
- ½ tablespoon lemon juice
- 1-2 teaspoons fresh tarragon leaves, torn, to garnish

Directions

1. Place the fully cooked grilled chicken strips in a skillet over medium-high heat and cook 3-5 minutes or until strips are heated through. Remove chicken from heat and set aside.
2. Wipe out the skillet and place it over medium heat. Add in ½ tablespoon coconut oil and allow it to heat up. Add in the chopped garlic; sauté 1 to 2 minutes or until fragrant. Add in the sliced fennel, season with 1 teaspoon sea salt, or to taste. Sauté for 2 to 3 minutes or until the fennel is slightly softened.
3. Add in the sliced radicchio; season again with ½ teaspoon sea salt, or to taste. Sauté 1 to 2 minutes more or until radicchio begins wilting and turning brown in spots. Remove from heat immediately and add a splash of lemon juice.
4. To serve, place the radicchio/fennel salad mixture on a serving plate and top the grilled chicken strips, and a few of the torn tarragon leaves. Finally, drizzle the salad with red wine vinegar; season with additional sea salt, if needed, to taste, then serve immediately.

Nutritional Data

- Calories: 289
- Total Fat: 7
- Carbohydrates: 27
- Fiber: 7
- Sugars: 7
- Protein: 24

Lunch Recipe: Chicken Curry Soup with Coconut and Lime

- Servings: 1 (serving size: 1½ to 2 cups soup)
- Total time (prep to finish): 20 minutes

Ingredients

- 1 cup reduced-sodium chicken broth
- ¼ cup unsweetened coconut milk
- ¼ tablespoon curry powder
- ½ jalapeno pepper, seeded and minced

- 6-8 ounces boneless skinless chicken breast halves, cut into ¾-inch cubes
- 1 tablespoon fresh lime juice
- ¼ teaspoon sea salt, or to taste
- ¼ teaspoon fresh ground black pepper, or to taste
- ½ cup green onion (white and green parts), chopped
- ½ cup fresh cilantro, chopped
- 1 cup cauliflower, riced and steamed
- 2 lime wedges, to serve

Directions

1. Rice the cauliflower and steam until tender and heated through.
2. Meanwhile, bring the chicken broth, coconut milk, curry powder and the jalapeno to a simmer in a heavy medium saucepan over medium heat.
3. Add chicken and simmer for about 5 minutes or until chicken is just cooked through, stirring frequently. Stir in the lime juice and season to taste with sea salt and fresh ground black pepper.
4. Place the cauliflower rice in a serving bowl. Ladle the soup over the rice.
5. To serve, garnish with chopped green onion and fresh cilantro. Season with additional salt and pepper, if needed, to taste and serve with 2 wedges of lime.

Nutritional Data

- Calories: 236
- Total Fat: 7
- Carbohydrates: 14
- Fiber: 5
- Sugars: 5
- Protein: 28

....

Dinner

Dinner Recipe:

Baked Chicken and Sautéed Brussels Sprouts

- Servings: 2 (serving size: 6 ounces chicken; 1½ cups sautéed Brussels sprouts)
- Total time (prep to finish): 55 minutes

Ingredients

- 2 (4-6 ounces) free-range boneless, skinless chicken breasts
- 4 tablespoons extra-virgin olive oil, divided

- 2 tablespoons lemon juice, divided
- ½ teaspoon salt, or to taste, divided
- ¼ teaspoon fresh ground black pepper, divided
- ⅛-¼ teaspoon tarragon (optional)
- 1 teaspoon dried parsley, divided
- 4 cups small Brussels sprouts
- 1 tablespoon extra-virgin olive oil (plus more for rubbing)
- ⅛ teaspoon fresh ground black pepper (to taste)
- ¼ teaspoon sea salt (to taste)
- ¼ cup preferred raw cheese, finely grated

Directions

1. Preheat oven to 350°F. Rinse the chicken breasts in cool running water; cut off any visible excess fat, and place the chicken breasts in a baking dish. Season the chicken with sea salt, black pepper, and the tarragon (optional). Drizzle ½ tablespoon lemon juice and ½ tablespoon olive oil over each chicken breast. Then top each breast with ½ teaspoon dried parsley, and ½ tablespoon more of lemon juice.

2. Place the chicken in the preheated oven, and bake for 35-40 minutes or until the chicken is cooked through and juices run clear (the chicken should reach an internal temperature of 165°F).

3. When the chicken is nearly finished baking, prepare the Brussels sprouts. Wash the sprouts well, and remove and discard any outer leaves.

4. Slice each sprout in half lengthwise from the stem to the top of the sprout, then brush the halves with 3 tablespoons of the olive oil, or as needed.

5. Place a large sauté pan over medium heat. Add in the remaining 1 tablespoon olive oil, and allow it a couple of minutes to heat up just a little, then lay the Brussels sprouts in the pan, flat half facing down.

6. Sprinkle the sprouts with sea salt and black pepper. Allow the sprouts to sauté, moving the sprouts around, so they do not stick to the pan.

7. Sauté 3 to 5 minutes or until the flat side of the sprouts turns lightly golden brown and is fork-tender. (Make sure you can pierce the fork completely through the sprouts.)

8. Once fork tender, turn up the heat to high, and cook for 2 to 4 minutes or just long enough for the flat sides of the sprouts to become caramelized and a deep golden brown. Then begin tossing/stirring and moving the sprouts around to gain a little bit of browning on the rounded sides as well.

9. Transfer 1½ cups to a serving dish, and sprinkle on a bit more sea salt and black pepper, if needed, and then finally, sprinkle the finely raw

grated cheese over the sprouts. Serve alongside the baked chicken and enjoy!

10. Let the remaining chicken and sprouts cool completely at room temperature. Then store in sealable containers in the refrigerator to serve as lunch the following day. When ready to serve, just remove from refrigerator and reheat!

Nutritional Data

- Calories: 415
- Total Fat: 44
- Carbohydrates: 15
- Fiber: 6
- Protein: 32

Dinner Recipe:
Spiced Steak with Grilled Pepper Salad

This is another Cost-Conscious Meal—less than $4.50 per serving. A dish originally prepared for lunch, which makes an excellent and very inexpensive side dish!

- Servings: 4 (serving size: one 4-6 ounces grilled sirloin steak; 1½ cups salad)
- Total time (prep to finish): 35 minutes

Ingredients

- 6 grass-fed sirloin steaks (4-6 ounces each; New York cut or preferred cut), all visible fat trimmed
- 2⅔ tablespoons white wine vinegar
- 4 large garlic cloves, crushed
- 1⅓ tablespoons water
- 1⅓ tablespoons ground coriander
- 2 teaspoons ground cumin
- 2 teaspoons chili powder
- 4 bell peppers, (red, yellow, green, orange), stems/seeds discarded, halved
- ¼ cup oil-cured black olives, pitted and halved
- ¼ cup sun-dried tomatoes, rinsed/chopped
- 1-2 tablespoons extra-virgin olive oil
- 1-2 tablespoons balsamic vinegar
- ⅛-¼ teaspoon sea salt, to taste
- ⅛-¼ cup raw feta or goat cheese, crumbled

Directions

1. Use a sharp knife to very lightly score both sides of the steak in a diamond pattern. In a small bowl, combine the white wine vinegar with

the garlic, water, coriander, cumin, and chili powder, and mix well. Use a pastry brush to brush the mixture evenly over both sides of each steak. Place steaks on a plate, covered, in the fridge for 15 minutes to marinate.

2. Preheat a barbecue grill on medium-high. Place the bell pepper halves, face down, on the grill, and cook for 4-5 minutes or until nicely charred. Turn the peppers over, and continue grilling for 4-5 minutes more or until the peppers are nicely charred. Remove from grill, and transfer to a cutting board.

3. Next, place the steaks on the grill, and cook for 5-7 minutes per side for medium or until cooked to your liking. While the steaks are grilling, prepare the side salad.

4. First, when the grilled peppers are cool enough to handle, chop them up into bite-sized pieces. Place the chopped bell peppers in a large salad bowl. Add in the halved olives, chopped sun-dried tomatoes, olive oil, vinegar, sea salt, and raw crumbled cheese, and toss/stir to mix well.

5. Serve one of the steaks alongside 1½ cups of the grilled pepper salad. Reserve the remaining steaks and salad to be used as directed throughout the 30-day meal plan.

Nutritional Data
- Calories: 355
- Total Fat: 18
- Carbohydrates: 10
- Fiber: 4
- Protein: 37

Dinner Recipe:
Steak and Asparagus Stir-Fry
- Servings: 4 (serving size: 2 cups stir-fry)
- Total time (prep to finish): 20 minutes

Ingredients
- 2 tablespoons coconut oil
- 2 pounds asparagus, trimmed and cut diagonally into 1½-inch lengths, to yield 8 cups
- 4 (4-6 ounces each) grass-fed steaks (preferred cut), grilled and sliced into thin strips
- 2-3 teaspoons fresh ginger, peeled and finely chopped
- 4 small cloves of garlic, minced
- 4 green onions (white and green parts), sliced, divided
- 4 tablespoons sesame seeds, toasted, to garnish (optional)

Directions

1. Bring a Dutch oven or large stockpot of water to a boil. While waiting for water to boil, prepare the ingredients as directed. When water begins to boil, add the asparagus pieces and parboil for 2 minutes, then drain and rinse in cold water. Drain again, and set aside.

2. Place a wok over medium-high heat. Add in 1 tablespoon coconut oil, and allow it to heat up. Add the asparagus and stir-fry in for about 2 minutes or until lightly browned. Remove asparagus from wok; set aside.

3. Add another 1 tablespoon coconut oil to wok. Let it heat. Then add in the steak strips in a single layer, followed by the chopped ginger, minced garlic, and green onions. Stir to mix well. Stir-fry for 5-7 minutes or until the steak is cooked through. Return the asparagus to the wok, and toss to mix with other ingredients.

4. Transfer 2 cups of the stir-fry to a serving dish and garnish with 1 tablespoon toasted sesame seeds, if desired, and then serve and enjoy!

5. Divide the remaining 6 cups steak-asparagus stir-fry into 2-cup portions in separate sealable containers, and store in the freezer to be used as directed throughout the 30-day meal plan. When ready to use, just reheat and serve!

Nutritional Data

- Calories: 496
- Total Fat: 15
- Carbohydrates: 13
- Fiber: 6
- Protein: 33

....

Dinner Recipe:
Grilled Salmon, Zucchini and Broccoli Salad

- Servings: 4 (serving size: 1 (6-ounce) salmon portion; 2 spears zucchini; 1½ cups salad)
- Total time (prep to finish): 30 minutes

Ingredients

- 1 zucchini, cut into 4 spears
- 2 tablespoons extra-virgin olive oil, divided
- ¼ teaspoon sea salt, or to taste, divided
- ⅛ teaspoon fresh ground black pepper, or to taste
- 2½ cloves garlic, minced, divided
- 2 (6 ounces) wild salmon fillets
- ½-1 tablespoon fresh basil, chopped

- ¼ cup raw milk feta goat cheese, crumbled
- ¼-½ cup organic whole or goat's milk plain yogurt
- 1-2 tablespoons lemon juice
- 3 cups broccoli florets, trimmed/chopped
- ¼ purple onion, sliced into thin rounds and halved
- ½-1 cup red bell pepper, chopped

Directions

1. Preheat grill to medium-high heat.
2. Place the zucchini spears in a bowl with 1 tablespoon olive oil (or more as needed to evenly coat), ⅛ teaspoon sea salt, and 1/16 teaspoon black pepper. Toss to coat the zucchini in the oil and seasonings.
3. Mash ½ clove of the minced garlic and ⅛ teaspoon of the salt on a cutting board with the side of a chef's knife or a spoon until a paste forms. Transfer to a small bowl, and stir in the remaining 1 tablespoon olive oil.
4. Check the salmon for any pin bones; remove and discard. Measure out a piece of heavy-duty aluminum foil (or a double layer of regular foil) large enough for each salmon fillet. Coat the foil with cooking spray. Place the salmon skin-side-down on each piece of foil, and spread the garlic mixture all over it. Sprinkle each salmon fillet with some of the fresh basil.
5. Transfer the salmon fillets on the foils to the grill. Grill for 10-12 minutes or until the salmon flakes easily and reaches an internal temperature of 145°F.
6. While the salmon is grilling, prepare the broccoli salad. In a large-sized mixing bowl, combine the raw crumbled cheese, the yogurt, the remaining 1-2 cloves of minced garlic, lemon juice, and a pinch of the black pepper. Whisk until smooth and well blended. Prepare the broccoli, purple onion, and bell pepper as directed. Then add them to the yogurt dressing. Toss/stir to mix, and coat the salad contents well with the yogurt dressing. Salad can be served chilled or at room temperature.
7. Using two large spatulas, slide one of the salmon fillets onto a serving plate, and serve alongside 2 spears of zucchini and the broccoli salad.
8. Store the remaining salmon fillets, zucchini, and broccoli salad in the refrigerator/freezer in sealable containers to be used as directed throughout 30-day meal plan.
9. To grill the zucchini, place the slices directly on the grill. Let grill for 5-6 minutes, and then flip the slices and grill for an additional 5-6 minutes or until fork-tender. If you want crisscross grill marks, rotate each piece halfway through cooking on both sides.
10. To serve, place the remaining salmon fillet on a serving plate alongside

1½-2 cups of the grilled zucchini slices. Sprinkle the salmon fillet with a little of the remaining basil and serve.

Nutritional Data
- Calories: 347
- Total Fat: 32
- Carbohydrates: 29
- Fiber: 9
- Protein: 46

Dinner Recipe:
Char-grilled Chicken, Roasted Broccoli, and Baby Spinach Salad

This Cost-Conscious Meal costs less than $3.75 per serving when using the grill and combining with fresh vegetables such as broccoli, asparagus, Brussels sprouts, fresh greens, etc.

- Servings: 2 (serving size: six ounces chicken; 2 cups broccoli; 1½ cups salad); 6 extra breasts are grilled to store and use for other meals on the 30-day meal plan)
- Total time (prep to finish): 55 minutes

Ingredients
- 8 free-range boneless, skinless chicken breasts (6 ounces each)
- Zest from 1 lime, finely grated
- Juice from 4-6 limes
- 4-6 tablespoons extra virgin olive oil, divided
- 3 cloves garlic, crushed
- 4 cups raw broccoli, broken into florets
- ⅛-¼ teaspoon sea salt
- ⅛ teaspoon fresh ground black pepper
- 3 cups baby spinach, torn
- ¼ cup cucumber, sliced
- ⅛ cup red onion, chopped
- 2 tablespoons vegan dressing of choice

Directions
1. Begin by roasting the broccoli: Preheat the oven to 425°F. Line a rimmed baking sheet with aluminum foil.
2. Place the broccoli on the foil-lined baking sheet. Drizzle with 1-2 tablespoon of the olive oil, and then sprinkle on the sea salt and black pepper.
3. Place in the middle of the preheated oven, and roast for 40-45 minutes or until the stems of the broccoli are fork tender. Toward the last 10 minutes or so, keep a watchful eye on the roasting broccoli as the

florets can go from perfectly browned to black in a matter of a few minutes.

4. As soon as the broccoli is put in the oven to roast, begin grilling the chicken breasts, as you have to account for marinating time. Cut any excess/visible fat from the chicken breasts, and rinse the chicken breasts in cool running water. Pat dry with paper towels.

5. Prepare the marinade by combining the lime zest, lime juice, the remaining 2-4 tablespoons olive oil, and the crushed garlic into a shallow glass bowl. Whisk until the contents are well incorporated, adding a little more olive oil, if needed.

6. Place the chicken breasts in the marinade, turning to coat each breast with the marinade as best as possible. Cover the bowl with plastic wrap, and place in the refrigerator for at least 15 minutes to marinate. Tip: You could also combine the marinade in a doubled gallon-sized Ziploc bag, and place the chicken breasts in the bag to marinate. Doing this can often make it easier to coat each piece with the marinade. If you are worried about the bag leaking, just lay the bag in a large bowl or in a shallow dish such as a pie pan to catch any leakage.

7. Preheat the grill. Place the chicken breasts on the grill, and grill for about 4-5 minutes per side or until nicely charred and cooked through. The chicken should reach an internal temperature of 165°F. Remove the chicken from the grill, and allow to cool for 5 minutes.

8. While the chicken breasts are grilling, prepare the salad. Place the torn baby spinach, sliced cucumber, and chopped red onion into a large salad bowl. Toss to mix. Drizzle on the vegan salad dressing of choice and toss to coat. Set aside in the refrigerator until needed.

9. Place one of the char-grilled breasts on a serving plate alongside the 2 cups of the roasted broccoli and 1½ cups of the prepared side salad. Serve immediately.

10. For the remaining 7 chicken breasts, place one of the breasts in a storage container, and store in the refrigerator to be used for the next day's lunch. Place the remaining 6 char-grilled chicken breasts in freezer wrap/freezer safe containers—individually—to be pulled out and reheated as directed throughout the 30-day meal plan. Allow the chicken breasts to cool completely at room temperature before placing in the freezer.

Nutritional Data

- Calories: 479
- Total Fat: 43
- Carbohydrates: 24
- Fiber: 11
- Protein: 42

Dinner Recipe:
Baked Basil Chicken over Fresh Greens with Asparagus

- Servings: 2 (serving size: 4-6 ounces baked chicken; 1½ cups fresh greens; ½ pound asparagus spears)
- Total time (prep to finish): 45 minutes

Ingredients

- 2 boneless, skinless chicken breast halves (¾ pound, approximately 4-6 ounces each)
- 1 pound asparagus spears
- 2 green onions (both white and green parts), chopped
- ⅛ cup extra-virgin olive oil
- 1 tablespoon white wine vinegar
- 1 teaspoon fresh ginger, chopped fine
- 1 tablespoon fresh basil, chopped fine (or 1-2 teaspoons dried basil)
- 3 cups fresh spinach (or fresh greens of choice)

Directions

1. Rinse the chicken breasts in cool, running water; pat dry using paper towel. Cut away any visible or excess fat.
2. In a medium-size glass bowl, combine the green onion, olive oil, vinegar, fresh ginger, and fresh (or dried) basil; whisk together to create the marinade.
3. Arrange the chicken breasts in a shallow baking dish, and pour the marinade over the chicken, turning to coat. Cover with plastic wrap, and place the marinating chicken in the refrigerator for 30 minutes.
4. Preheat oven to 375°F. Line a rimmed baking sheet with aluminum foil. Place the chicken breasts on the foil-lined baking sheet, and arrange the rinsed/dried asparagus spears around the chicken breasts. Place the baking sheet in the preheated oven. Bake the chicken/asparagus for 35-45 minutes or until the asparagus is fork tender and the chicken breasts are cooked through and juices run clear.
5. To serve, place a baked chicken breast on each plate, and serve over a bed of fresh spinach or preferred greens and serve alongside 3-4 spears of asparagus.
6. Store the remaining Chicken/Greens/Asparagus in the sealable containers to be used for lunch the following day.

Nutritional Data

- Calories: 488
- Total Fat: 29
- Carbohydrates: 25

- Fiber: 13
- Protein: 39

Dinner Recipe:
Broiled Tilapia and Steamed Veggies
- Servings: 3 (serving size: 4 to 6 ounce tilapia fillet;
  1½-2 cups vegetables of choice)
- Total time (prep to finish): 20 minutes

Ingredients
- 3 wild caught tilapia fillets (4-6 ounces each)
- Sea salt (to taste)
- Fresh ground black pepper (to taste)
- 1 teaspoon dried oregano
- 1 teaspoon dried parsley
- 3 teaspoons extra-virgin olive oil, divided
- 1 clove fresh garlic, minced
- 1½-2 cups steamed or roasted vegetables of choice per serving

Directions
1. To prepare, turn on the broiler to low and preheat. Align an oven rack
   in the upper half of the oven about 8 inches from the broiler flame.
   Line a broiler pan with aluminum foil.
2. Rinse the tilapia fillets and pat dry. Then lay the tilapia on the foil-lined
   broiler pan, and season the fillets with the sea salt and black pepper, to
   taste, followed by the dried oregano and dried parsley.
3. Drizzle each fillet with 1 teaspoon olive oil, and then sprinkle on a
   pinch of the fresh minced garlic.
4. Place the broiler pan holding the tilapia fillets in the oven, and cook for
   5-7 minutes or until the fish is cooked through.
5. Remove from broiler, and immediately splash the fillets with lemon
   juice.
6. Transfer one of the tilapia fillets to a serving dish, and serve alongside
   steamed or roasted vegetables of choice.
7. Store the remaining fillets individually in freezer wrap, and store the
   wrapped fillets in the freezer to be used as directed throughout the 30-
   day meal plan.

Nutritional Data
- Calories: 390
- Total Fat: 12
- Carbohydrates: 23
- Fiber: 10
- Protein: 52

Dinner Recipe:
Barbecued Sirloin in Dijon Dressing with Grilled Vegetables
- Servings: 4 (serving size: 4-6 ounces sirloin steak; ¼ cup Dijon dressing; 2 cups grilled mixed vegetables)
- Total time (prep to finish): 30 minutes

Ingredients
- 4 grass-fed beef sirloin steaks (4-6 ounces each)
- 2 tablespoons fresh basil, coarsely chopped
- 2 teaspoons fresh ground black pepper
- 2 tablespoons Dijon mustard
- 2 tablespoons olive oil
- 2 tablespoons white wine vinegar
- 8 cups grilled mixed vegetables

Directions
1. In a bowl, combine the basil, the black pepper, the olive oil, the Dijon mustard and the white wine vinegar.
2. Rub the marinade onto the sirloin steaks, and refrigerate for at least 15 minutes to marinate.
3. Preheat the grill to medium-high, and cook the steak 5-7 minutes per side or until desired doneness is reached. Meanwhile, grill chosen vegetables until heated through.
4. Let the meat rest around 5-10 minutes before serving. Serve alongside 2 cups grilled vegetables.

Nutritional Data
- Calories: 251
- Total Fat: 7
- Carbohydrates: 10
- Fiber: 4
- Protein: 53

Dinner Recipe:
Black Bean Chili
- Servings: 8 (Serving Size: 1½-2 cups chili)
- Total Time (prep to finish): 30 minutes

Ingredients
- 2 pounds organic ground turkey (or grass-fed ground beef, if preferred)
- 2-3 cans gluten-free black beans, rinsed/drained
- 1 large white onion(s), diced

- 1 green bell pepper, chopped (optional)
- 3-4 (14-oz.) cans diced tomatoes
- ½ cup water
- 2-4 tablespoons chili powder, to taste
- Desired toppings: raw shredded cheese, sliced green onions, etc.

Directions

1. Place a Dutch oven or a deep, heavy-bottomed pan over medium heat. Add in the ground turkey (or beef) and cook, stirring occasionally to help crumble up the meat for 6-8 minutes or until browned. Drain, then return meat to the Dutch oven/pan.
2. Add in the onion and bell pepper, and cook for 2-3 minutes, mixing the veggies with the ground meat, until the onion and pepper are fork tender. Sprinkle in the desired amount of chili powder; stir to incorporate.
3. Next, add in the water, black beans, and diced tomatoes, and stir to incorporate. Then allow the contents to come to a boil, stirring occasionally. Once the chili begins to boil, reduce heat to low, cover and simmer for 20 minutes, stirring occasionally. Then uncover and continue cooking an additional 5 minutes more.
4. Ladle 1½ to 2 cups of chili into a bowl, top with desired toppings, and enjoy.
5. Let the remaining chili cool completely. Then using sealable storage containers, store the remaining chili in separate 1½-2 cups portions to be pulled out and reheated as directed throughout 30-day meal plan.

Nutritional Data

- Calories: 350
- Total Fat: 14
- Carbohydrates: 21
- Fiber: 7
- Protein: 39

Dinner Recipe:
Mediterranean Stew

- Servings: 8 (serving size 1½ to 2 cups stew)
- Total time (prep to finish): 1 hour, 45 minutes

Ingredients

- 2 pounds grass-fed beef sirloin, cut into 1-inch pieces (or use precut stew meat).
- 1-2 tablespoons coconut oil
- 1 cup button mushrooms, sliced
- 1 cup frozen pearl onions, thawed

- 4 cloves garlic, minced
- 3½ cups beef broth or stock, divided
- 3 (28 oz.) cans crushed tomatoes with juice
- 3 (6 oz.) cans tomato paste
- 1 tablespoon arrowroot powder
- 2 cups baby spinach, torn
- ⅛-¼ cup fresh basil, chopped
- ⅛-¼ cup fresh oregano, chopped
- 1 tablespoon sea salt, or to taste
- 1 tablespoon fresh ground black pepper, or to taste

Directions

1. Begin by preparing the beef, trim off any excess fat, and cut into 1-inch pieces. Season with sea salt and pepper. Place a Dutch oven or large pot over medium-high heat. Add in 1 tablespoon coconut oil, and let it heat up. Add the pieces of beef to the skillet, and brown it on all sides for 5 to 7 minutes. Transfer to plate, and set aside until needed.

2. In the Dutch oven/pot, now add in ½ tablespoon coconut oil, and let melt; then combine the sliced button mushrooms, pearl onions, and garlic, and sauté for 5 minutes, stirring often. Place the browned meat back into the Dutch oven/pot, and stir to combine the contents. Add in 3 cups beef broth (or stock), cans of crushed tomatoes (plus juices), tomato paste, and a little water, if needed, to thin. Bring contents to a boil. Then reduce heat to medium, cover and simmer for 45 minutes.

3. In a small bowl, whisk together the remaining ½ cup broth (or stock), and 1-2 tablespoons arrowroot powder, depending on thickness desired. Then stir the mixture into the stew after 45 minutes, along with adding in the baby spinach, fresh basil, and the fresh oregano. Stir with wooden spoon to mix well. Sprinkle in the sea salt and black pepper, and stir to incorporate.

4. Cook for an additional 20-30 minutes or until the beef is cooked through, the onions are fork tender, and the spinach is nicely wilted. Taste, and adjust seasonings as necessary. Note: you can also make this stew by combining all ingredients into a slow cooker, and cooking on low heat for 7 hours or on high heat for 3-4 hours.

5. Ladle 1½ to 2 cups stew per serving bowl, and serve. Let the remaining stew cool completely. Then using sealable storage containers, store the remaining stew in separate 1½ to 2 cups portions to be pulled out and reheated as directed throughout 30-day meal plan.

Nutritional Data

- Calories: 329
- Total Fat: 6

- Carbohydrates: 40
- Fiber: 8
- Protein: 37

....

Dinner Recipe:
Eggplant Ratatouille
- Servings: 1 (serving size: 1½ to 2 cups)
- Total time (prep to finish): 10 minutes

Ingredients
- ½ tablespoon coconut oil
- ½ small white onion, thinly sliced
- ½ red bell pepper, thinly sliced
- 1 clove garlic, crushed
- ¼ small eggplant, chopped
- ½ small zucchini, sliced diagonally
- 1½ tablespoons red wine vinegar
- ½ large tomato, chopped
- ¼ cup cold water
- ¼ teaspoon sea salt, to taste
- ⅛ teaspoon fresh ground black pepper, to taste

Directions
1. Place the coconut oil in a Dutch oven or a large, heavy-bottomed saucepan. Let the oil heat up over medium-high heat. Add in the red bell pepper and onion. Sauté for 2 minutes or until softened. Add garlic and sauté for one minute.
2. While the pepper/onion is sautéing, chop up the eggplant and slice the zucchini, diagonally, into rounds. Add the eggplant and zucchini to the pepper/onion and stir to combine. Let sauté for 2 more minutes or just until just softened.
3. Next, add in the vinegar and chopped tomato. Cook for 30 seconds, stirring constantly, until the vinegar has evaporated. Add in ¼ cup cold water, season with salt and black pepper and bring to a simmer. Allow the ratatouille to simmer, covered, for 4 minutes or until the sauce has thickened and the vegetables are fork-tender.
4. Place 1½-2 cups ratatouille on a serving plate and enjoy!

Nutritional Data
- Calories: 147
- Total Fat: 12
- Carbohydrates: 11
- Fiber: 2
- Protein: 4

Snacks and Desserts

Snack/Dessert Recipe:
Chocolate-Avocado Brownies with Walnuts
- Servings: 12 (serving size: 1 brownie)
- Total time (prep to finish): 1½ hours

Ingredients
- ¾ cup almond meal
- ¼ cup unsweetened cocoa powder
- ½ teaspoon baking powder
- ½ teaspoon sea salt
- 3 tablespoons coconut oil
- 1 teaspoon vanilla extract
- 2 large pasture-raised eggs
- 2 large ripe avocados
- 8 ounces vegan/allergen-free dark chocolate—70% or higher—and chopped (Enjoy Life, Alter Eco, Kallari, etc.)
- 1 tablespoon Stevia powder extract (or 18-24 Stevia packets), or to taste
- ½ cup walnuts, chopped

Directions
1. Preheat oven to 350°F. Line an 8 x 8-inch baking pan with aluminum foil—enough so that the foil hangs over the sides of the pan. The overhanging foil will later act as handles, making it much easier to remove the brownies from the pan, in order to cut them.
2. To begin, place the chopped chocolate and coconut oil in a microwave-safe bowl and heat in 15-30 second intervals, stirring between each interval with a wooden spoon, until the coconut oil and chocolate are completely melted and smooth. Stir the mixture well to blend. Let the coconut oil-chocolate mixture rest at room temperature for 5 minutes.
3. Meanwhile, peel the avocados, remove/discard stones, and place the avocado flesh in a large mixing bowl. Mash the avocado until smooth. Next, stir the coconut oil-chocolate mixture in with the mashed avocado, and stir to blend. Next, stir in the Stevia powder extract (or packets) until completely incorporated. Then add the eggs—one at a time—then finally, stir in the vanilla extract.
4. In a separate bowl, first sift in the cocoa powder. Then stir in the almond meal, sea salt, and baking powder. Then add the dry mixture to the avocado mixture, and stir with a wooden spoon just until combined. Be sure to not over-mix. Fold in the walnuts, and then add the brownie batter to the prepared baking pan, and spread out to fill the pan,

smoothing the top of the batter with a rubber spatula.

5. Place the pan in the preheated oven, and bake for 25-28 minutes or until a toothpick inserted into the center of the brownies comes out clean. Remove from oven, and let the brownies cool in the pan for 10 minutes. Hold the foil on either side of the pan, and carefully lift the brownies out of the pan. Transfer the foil to a wire cooling rack, and allow the brownies to cool some more before slicing and serving. Store the remaining brownies in an airtight container at room temperature (or in the refrigerator, if preferred) until needed as directed throughout the 30-day meal plan.

Nutritional Data

- Calories: 298
- Total Fat: 25
- Carbohydrates: 25
- Fiber: 1
- Protein: 21

Snack/Dessert Recipe: Gooey Chocolate Chip Cookies

This Cost-Conscious recipe makes 3 dozen cookies for less than $5, as it uses many ingredients remaining from other dishes that are common pantry items, such as leftover coconut and almond flours, grass-fed butter, stevia, eggs, etc. Bonus: these cookies store amazingly well in the freezer so just pull some out when ready to serve!

- Servings: 18 (serving size: 2 cookies)
- Total Time (prep to finish): 45 minutes

Ingredients

- 3 cups blanched almond flour
- 1 tablespoon coconut flour
- 1 teaspoon sea salt
- ¾ teaspoon baking soda
- ½ teaspoon baking powder
- ½ cup grass-fed butter, melted
- ¼ tablespoon Stevia powder extract (or 8-10 Stevia packets)
- ½-1 teaspoon Xylitol
- 2 large pasture-raised eggs, room temperature
- 1½ tablespoons pure vanilla extract
- 1 (10 ounces) package vegan semi-sweet chocolate chips (Enjoy Life or preferred brand)

Directions

1. Combine the blanched almond flour, coconut flour, salt, baking soda,

and baking powder and whisk until well blended; set aside.

2. In a food processor, combine melted grass-fed butter and Stevia. Process mixture for one minute or until the contents are blended well. Next, add in the Xylitol, eggs, and vanilla extract. Process until smooth and creamy. Add the flour mixture, and process in food processor, until dough is completely blended and smooth.

3. Transfer the dough to a mixing bowl, and then fold in the chocolate chips, using a wooden spoon. When the chocolate chips are well incorporated, set the cookie dough aside to rest, at room temperature, for 15 minutes. The dough will become more solid and easier to work with as it rests.

4. Preheat the oven to 350°F. Arrange the oven racks in center of oven. Line 2-3 baking sheets with parchment paper. Using a tablespoon, scoop out a rounded tablespoon of the dough, and drop it onto the parchment-lined baking sheet. Repeat until all the dough has been used up, placing them about 1-2 inches apart on the baking sheets. Yields about 36 cookies.

5. Place the cookies in the oven, and bake for 10-12 minutes or until the edges/bottom of the cookies are golden brown and the centers appear slightly uncooked, puffy, and lightly crackled. Be careful not to let the cookies bake for more than 12 minutes, or they will become too dry and hard.

6. Remove the cookies from the oven, and let cool for 5-10 minutes on the baking sheets. Then transfer to wire racks to cool completely. Serve cookies immediately, or keep them stored in an airtight container at room temperature or in the freezer.

Nutritional Data
- Calories: 124
- Total Fat: 9
- Carbohydrates: 4
- Fiber: 2
- Protein: 5

Snack/Dessert Recipe: Chocolate-Dipped Macaroons
- Servings: 10 (serving size: 2 cookies)
- Total Time (prep to finish): 1 hour, 35 minutes
  (inactive: 1 hour chill time)

Ingredients
- 8 large pasture-raised egg whites
- ½ tablespoon Stevia powder extract (or 9-12 Stevia packets)

- 4 cups unsweetened shredded coconut
- 4 tablespoons coconut flour
- 2 teaspoons almond extract
- ¼ teaspoon sea salt (to taste)
- 12-16 ounces vegan semisweet or dark chocolate chips

Directions

1. Preheat oven to 325°F. Line 2 baking sheets with parchment paper.
2. In a large mixing bowl, whisk the egg whites, Stevia, almond extract, and salt.
3. Then add in the coconut and flour, and mix until well incorporated.
4. Set in the refrigerator for 1 hour to harden.
5. Scoop the dough into 1-inch semi-rolled pieces, and lay the pieces on the parchment-lined baking sheet. Bake for 18-20 minutes or until the macaroons are lightly toasted and the bottom edges are golden brown. Remove from oven, and let cool completely.
6. Melt the chocolate chips in the microwave or double boiler. Dip the top of each macaroon in chocolate and place the dipped macaroons on a sheet of parchment or wax paper to set. Let the chocolate harden at room temperature or in the refrigerator. Once the chocolate is firm, serve and enjoy!

Nutritional Data

- Calories: 250
- Total Fat: 16
- Carbohydrates: 27
- Fiber: 3
- Protein: 4

Snack/Dessert Recipe: Crispy Butterscotch Cookies

Cost-Conscious Meal: Cookies make excellent budget-friendly treats since they usually use common ingredients found in most household pantries. One batch typically yields a large number of cookies, enabling you to freeze some and store some in airtight containers at room temperature for quick treats anytime!

- Servings: 12 (serving size: 2 cookies)
- Total time (prep to finish): 25 minutes

Ingredients

- 2 cups almond flour
- ¼ cup coconut oil
- ¼ tablespoon Stevia extract powder (or ¼ teaspoon liquid Stevia or 5-6 Stevia packets)
- ½-1 teaspoon Xylitol

- ½ teaspoon butterscotch extract
- ¼ teaspoon sea salt

Directions

1. Preheat oven to 350°F. Line a baking sheet with parchment paper.
2. In a medium mixing bowl, mix together the almond flour, coconut oil, Stevia, Xylitol, butterscotch extract, and sea salt until a nice dough forms.
3. Form 1-inch balls with the dough, and place the dough balls on the parchment-lined baking sheet. You should have enough dough to make 24 balls.
4. Flatten cookies gently by stamping with a fork. Once with the fork tines straight up and down and once side-to-side. You will make a cross shape with your fork.
5. Place in the preheated oven and bake 8 to 10 minutes or until lightly browned around the edges. Remove from oven, let cool for at least 5 minutes before serving.

Nutritional Data

- Calories: 88
- Total Fat: 9
- Carbohydrates: 7
- Fiber: 1
- Protein: 1

....

Snack/Dessert Recipe: Almond Butter "Granola" Bars

- Servings: 14 (serving size: 1 bar)
- Total time (prep to finish): 15 minutes

Ingredients

- 1½ cups almond butter
- 1½ cups white sesame seeds
- 1-2 tablespoons Xylitol
- ½ cup unsweetened flaked coconut
- ½ cup sunflower seeds OR pumpkin seeds
- ½ cup walnuts, chopped fine
- ½ cup pecans, chopped fine
- Stevia, to taste
- 2 teaspoons cinnamon
- 1 teaspoon vanilla extract
- ⅛ teaspoon sea salt

Directions

1. Preheat oven to 350°F. In a large mixing bowl, combine the almond butter, Xylitol, Stevia, cinnamon, vanilla extract, and sea salt. Mix until well blended.
2. Next, add to the mixing bowl the shredded coconut, sesame seeds, and sunflower seeds (or pumpkin seeds). Blend together thoroughly.
3. In a food processor, chop walnuts and pecans, and then transfer the chopped nuts to the almond butter mixture. Blend well.
4. Press the mixture into a 9 X 11-inch baking dish, and bake for 9 to 11 minutes or until slightly browned.
5. Remove from heat, flip out onto a piece of parchment paper, and let cool completely before serving, storing, or freezing.

Nutritional Data

- Calories: 247
- Total Fat: 21
- Carbohydrates: 8
- Fiber: 2
- Protein: 8

Snack/Dessert Recipe:
Apple Nachos With Chocolate and Nut Toppings

- Servings: 1 (serving size: 1 apple with toppings)
- Total time (prep to finish): 10 minutes

Ingredients

- 1 large Granny Smith green apple, cut into wedges
- 1 to 2 tablespoons fresh lemon juice (more or less as needed to splash apple wedges)
- ¼ to ½ cup almond butter
- ¼ cup vegan chocolate chips, divided (such as Enjoy Life)
- ¼ cup unsweetened shredded coconut
- 1 to 2 tablespoons almonds, sliced

Directions

1. First, slice the apple and place the wedges in a bowl. Squeeze the lemon juice over the bowl and toss to coat.
2. Arrange the apple wedges on a dessert plate.
3. Using a pastry/piping bag or a Ziploc bag, drizzle the almond butter over the apple wedges.
4. Finally, sprinkle the dish with ¼ to ½ cup shredded coconut, ¼ to ½ cup chocolate chips, and 1 to 2 tablespoons sliced almonds. Serve and enjoy!

Nutritional Data
- Calories: 158
- Total Fat: 12
- Carbohydrates: 13
- Fiber: 2
- Protein: 3

....

Snack/Dessert Recipe: Yogurt Vegetable Dip
- Servings: 4 (serving size: ½ cup dip)
- Total time (prep to finish): 40 minutes

Ingredients
- 2 cups plain Greek or goat's milk yogurt
- 1 cup diced cucumber
- 2 tablespoons finely chopped fresh dill
- 2 tablespoons fresh lemon juice
- 2 cloves minced garlic
- Sea salt, to taste
- Fresh ground black pepper, to taste

Directions
1. Combine yogurt, cucumber, garlic, lemon juice, and dill. Add salt and pepper to taste.
2. Chill for at least 30 minutes before serving.

Nutritional Data
- Calories: 108
- Total Fat: 5
- Carbohydrates: 10
- Fiber: 0
- Protein: 7

....

Snack/Dessert Recipe: Green Smoothie
- Servings: 1 (serving size: 10 ounce green smoothie)
- Total time (prep to finish): 10 minutes

Ingredients
- 2 cups of kale, 1 head romaine lettuce, 2 cups spinach (or combination of the 3)
- ½ cup coconut milk
- 1 scoop Vanilla or Chocolate Perfect Protein
- 2 tablespoons cocoa powder
- ½ avocado

- 1 to 2 cups of crushed ice (depending on desired consistency)
- Stevia to taste

Directions

1. Put the lettuce, kale, and/or spinach in the blender with avocado and the coconut milk.
2. Blend until greens are fully mixed.
3. Add ice, cocoa powder, and Perfect Protein and mix until well blended.

Nutritional Data

- Calories: 577
- Total Fat: 43
- Carbohydrates: 33
- Fiber: 17
- Protein:

....

Snack/Dessert Recipe: Mixed Sweet Nuts

- Servings: 10 (serving size: ½ cup mixed nuts)
- Total time (prep to finish): 25 minutes

Ingredients

- 5 cups of raw, whole almonds, and/or pecans
- 1 large pasture-raised egg white
- 1 tablespoon of water
- ½ cup Xylitol
- 1 tablespoon cinnamon
- Pinch of salt

Directions

1. Mix together.
2. Cook for 15 minutes at 350°F degrees.
3. Stir and cook for another 10-15 minutes until browned.

Nutritional Data

- Calories: 299
- Total Fat: 35
- Carbohydrates: 19
- Fiber: 7
- Protein: 15

....

Snack/Dessert Recipe: Chocolate Malted Smoothie (1 serving)

- Total time (prep to finish): 10 minutes

Ingredients

- 1 cup coconut milk
- 1 to 2 cups of ice (depending on desired thickness and consistency)
- ½ avocado (makes it like a malt)
- 1 tablespoon of almond or peanut butter
- 2 to 3 tablespoons of unsweetened cocoa powder
- 1 scoop Chocolate Perfect Protein

Directions

1. Mix ingredients in a blender until desired consistency.
2. Enjoy!

Nutritional Data

- Calories: 478
- Total Fat: 39
- Carbohydrates: 20
- Fiber: 13
- Protein: 29

....

Snack/Dessert Recipe: Chocolate Chia Pudding (2 servings)

- Total time (prep to finish): 10 minutes

Ingredients

- 1 can of organic coconut milk
- 4 tablespoons of chia seeds
- 1.5 scoops of ML Chocolate Perfect Protein (Can make it pack even more of a protein punch with a tablespoon of organic, unsweetened cocoa powder and Stevia to taste)

Directions

1. Mix ingredients together until it makes a smooth solution with no clumps.
2. Refrigerate until it hardens.

Nutritional Data

- Calories: 359
- Total Fat: 29
- Carbohydrates: 9
- Fiber: 7
- Protein: 23

Snack/Dessert Recipe: Chocolate Avocado Pudding *(1 serving)*
- Total time (prep to finish): 10 minutes

Ingredients
- 1 avocado, soft and ripe, peeled and chopped
- 1 teaspoon vanilla
- ¼ cup cocoa powder
- Stevia to taste
- 6 tablespoons coconut milk (Or just water if cutting calories)
- ¼ cup of ice
- (Even better with a scoop of Perfect Protein)

Directions
1. Cut avocado in half, and remove pit. Scoop out flesh, and put in the blender along with remaining ingredients.
2. Process until smooth, occasionally scraping down sides. Serve immediately, or refrigerate until ready to serve. Ice keeps it from getting hot in the blender, so you can eat it right away.

Nutrition data (per serving)
- Calories: 580
- Total Fat: 47 (18 grams monounsaturated, 25 grams saturated, 4 grams polyunsaturated)
- Carbohydrates: 29
- Fiber: 16
- Protein: 10

Snack/Dessert Recipe:
Chocolate Almond Butter Fudge *(8 servings)*
- Total time (prep to finish): 2 hours 15 minutes

Ingredients
- 1 cup dark chocolate chips (73% dark)
- 1 cup almond butter
- 2 tablespoons Xylitol
- ½ tablespoon vanilla extract
- ¼ teaspoon sea salt

Directions
1. Melt chocolate in medium pot. Remove from heat, and stir in almond butter and Xylitol.
2. Once incorporated, stir in vanilla and salt.
3. Spread into a loaf pan, and refrigerate for at least 2 hours. Cut quickly

into small squares, and store in fridge or freezer. (Note: if using un-sweetened chocolate, use more Xylitol. If chocolate is less than 73% dark, eliminate Xylitol.)

Nutrition Data (per serving)

- Calories: 350
- Total Fat: 28 grams fat (16 grams monounsaturated, 7 grams saturated, 5 grams polyunsaturated)
- Carbohydrates: 18
- Fiber: 5
- Protein: 6

....

Snack/Dessert Recipe: Coconut Macaroons (12 macaroons)

- Total time (prep to finish): 40 minutes

Ingredients

- 1 cup organic raw almonds
- 2 cups unsweetened coconut flakes
- 1 scoop Maximized Living vanilla protein powder
- 3 tablespoons organic unsweetened cocoa
- Stevia or Xylitol to taste.
- 7 tablespoons warm (liquid) coconut oil
- 1 tablespoon flax seeds

Directions

1. In blender or food processor, grind almonds, flax seeds, and sesame seeds. Blend in remaining ingredients.
2. Remove mixture, and place tablespoon-sized macaroons on a cookie sheet or shallow baking dish and chill for at least 30 minutes.

Nutrition data (per macaroon)

- Calories: 200
- Total Fat: 17 grams fat (5 grams monounsaturated, 8 grams saturated, 2 grams polyunsaturated)
- Carbohydrates: 6
- Fiber: 3
- Protein: 15

Cost-Cutter Recipes by Chef Bryce Fluellen

Spice-Rubbed Sautéed Chicken, Apple, Blue-Cheese Crumbs and Balsamic Vinaigrette on a Bed of Mixed Greens

- Serves 6 to 8
- $2.00 per person

Main Ingredients

- 2 tablespoons olive oil
- 2 tablespoons spice rub (McCormick spice rub sold at local grocery store)
- 2 pounds skinless and boneless chicken breast or thigh meat (Use 1 pound for salad and save the rest for next day's lunch)
- 1 medium bowl of water (optional)
- 1 lemon (optional)
- 2 to 3 Granny Smith apples
- ½ cup of blue cheese crumbles
- 32 ounces of mixed greens or spinach

Vinaigrette Ingredients

- ½ cup of olive oil
- ¼ cup of balsamic vinegar
- 1 tablespoon of agave or other natural sweetener (honey)
- ¼ teaspoon of salt and pepper

Directions

1. Add ½ cup of olive oil to a mixing bowl, slowly mix in balsamic vinegar, and mix vigorously. Add salt and pepper and agave. Taste with spoon.
2. Core apples and slice into wedges. Place in bowl of water with squeeze of lemon to avoid browning.
3. Place chicken on cutting board and add rub on both sides.
4. Set bottom oven to 400 degrees. In a medium non-stick sautéing pan add two tablespoons of olive oil over medium heat. Add chicken and sauté about 5 to 7 minutes on each side until browned.
5. Place in the oven and finish cooking until the chicken reaches 160 degrees. This should be about 15 minutes depending on the oven. Once finished take it out of the oven and allow to rest about 5 minutes and then cut into squares.
6. Place mixed greens into a salad bowl and slowly add vinaigrette. Mix

lightly. Do not saturate the greens too heavily with dressing.

7. Toss in apple slices and blue cheese crumbs and mix gently. Add chicken pieces on the top.

Collard Green Salad

- 6 to 8 servings
- $1.00 per person

Ingredients

- 10-12 bunches of collard greens. Once cleaned and the stem is removed, roll up and cut length wise into bite size strips.
- 4 carrots. Remove the skin with a peeler (optional), and cut width-wise into half-inch circles.
- 8 ounces of button mushrooms. Cut width wise into slices.
- 8 ounces of strawberries (seasonal). Cut stem off and half.
- ¼ cup of seasoned rice vinegar
- 1 teaspoon of pepper
- 1 tablespoon of smoked or regular paprika
- ½ cup of olive oil

Directions

1. In a medium saucepan, bring cold water to boil over high heat. Add the collards and blanch for 2-3 minutes. We just want to remove some of the bitterness, but still keep the color and firmness.

2. Meanwhile, fill a large bowl with cold water and ice. When the collards are ready, drain them in colander, and then transfer to the cold water to stop cooking process. Once the collards are cooled, drain well and pat dry thoroughly with a paper towel.

3. Once complete, grab a large salad bowl and toss in the greens, carrots, and mushrooms. Mix the vinegar and olive oil together and add in pepper and smoked paprika. Mix half into the salad and massage thoroughly. Allow about 2-3 minutes for ingredients to combine. Add strawberries at the end and mix again.

4. Salad taste even better once allowed to sit overnight!

Mediterranean Three-Bean Salad

- 6 to 8 servings
- $1.00 per serving

Ingredients

- 1 can (15 ounces) white kidney beans
- 1 can (15 ounces) garbanzo beans
- 1 can (15 ounces) red kidney beans
- 1 medium size onion, diced
- 2 cloves garlic, minced
- 2 tablespoons of fresh parsley minced
- ½ cup of olive oil
- 2 lemons, juiced or ¼ cup of seasoned rice vinegar
- Salt & pepper to taste

Directions

1. Open and drain all cans of beans and toss in a medium size bowl.
2. Mix lemons or vinegar with olive oil.
3. Toss onion, garlic, and parsley in bowl with beans. Mix in dressing. Add salt and pepper.
4. Mix all ingredients and serve.

Core Cutter Recipes by Chef Bryce Fluellen

Quinoa Bean & Corn Salad

- 6 to 8 servings
- $1.75 per person

Dressing

- 3 tablespoons fresh lemon juice (juice of one small lemon)
- 2 tablespoons olive oil
- 2 tablespoons fresh cilantro or parsley, chopped
- 2 stalks scallions, chopped
- 1 teaspoon minced garlic
- 1 teaspoon cumin

Quinoa Mix

- 2 tablespoons fresh cilantro or parsley, chopped
- ¼ cup quinoa (rinsed under water) or bulgur
- ½ cup chicken or vegetable broth
- 1 can black beans, drained and rinsed
- 1 tomato, seeded and diced
- 1 cup fresh or frozen corn (use three ears if fresh corn)
- 1 pound cooked chicken saved from chicken salad

Directions

1. Cook quinoa or bulgur in broth for 12-15 minutes, until liquid is absorbed.
2. While grain cooks, mix dressing ingredients in a large bowl.
3. Add drained and rinsed beans, tomato and corn.
4. Cool grain to room temperature. Mix with dressing and chicken.
5. Chill until ready to eat.

Sweet Potato & Ginger Soup

- 4 to 6 servings
- $1.50 per person (estimated)

Ingredients

- 3 to 4 tablespoons of extra virgin olive oil
- 3 medium to large size sweet potatoes
- ½ cup of medium yellow or red onion, diced
- 1 leek diced, white only (optional)
- 32 ounces of low-sodium vegetable or chicken stock
- 1 tablespoon fresh ginger, skinned and chopped, or ½ tablespoon of dry
- 1 teaspoon of salt
- 1 teaspoon of black pepper
- 3 teaspoons of fresh thyme or 2 teaspoons of dry
- 1 tablespoon of fresh parsley
- 1 teaspoon of lemon

Directions

1. Roast sweet potatoes (Roasting brings out the natural sweetness) in the oven on 400 degrees until a fork goes right through potatoes (45-60 minutes).
2. Remove potatoes and allow to cool. Remove skin and place in a bowl.
3. Place medium size saucepot on stove burner and turn to medium heat. Add olive oil.
4. Once oil starts to shimmer add onion and ginger and sauté for about 5 minutes.
5. Toss in sweet potatoes, mash and mix in with onion and ginger.
6. Pour in full box of vegetable or chicken stock and turn pot on simmer and allow cooking for another 30 minutes.
7. Season with salt, pepper, and thyme. Grab hand mixer or place soup in blender and blend up soup until all ingredients are mixed well.

8. Chop up fresh parsley and place on top of the soup once ready to serve. Enjoy!

APPENDIX I

THOU SHALL EAT THIS	THOU SHALL NOT EAT THAT
Fruit—Good, Low Sugar Fruits: Raspberries, Blackberries, Blueberries, Strawberries Reduce High Sugar Fruits: Plums, Mangos, Figs, Oranges, Bananas, Grapes, Cherries	Concentrated fruit juice, preservative-filled dried fruit
Grains **(Eliminate on the Advanced Plan)**: Ancient grains: Amaranth, Quinoa, Millet, Oatmeal (Gluten free), Whole grain rice	Gluten foods: Wheat, Rye, Barley, White rice, Bread, Pasta
FLOUR - Almond Flour	White, Wheat, Rye, Barley flour
Vegetables, Veggie-Like & Starches: Broccoli, Asparagus, Eggplant, Green beans, Brussels sprouts, Peppers, Onion, Celery, Cucumber, Spinach, Lettuce, Kale, Squash, Zucchini, Snow peas, Mushrooms, Cauliflower, Tomato, Avocado, Sweet Potato (great for recovery)	Corn, Potatoes
Legumes, Seeds and Nuts: Legumes (Beans, Lentils, Peanuts, and Peas), Raw nuts, Seeds, Nut flour, Chia, flax are best, Sunflower, pumpkin (To make these foods better and safer to consume, follow the soaking instructions found in Appendix IV, page 134.)	Nuts and seeds roasted in vegetable oil. No soy, soy protein, or soy milk. Common GMO foods: soy, canola, sugar beets, corn, wheat, tomatoes, and potatoes.
Sweeteners: Stevia (in moderation): Use on Core Plan or for Exercise Recovery; raw honey, organic maple syrup, and coconut sugar. Xylitol, Erythritol Malitol, Mannitol, and Sorbitol	Sucralose (Splenda), Aspartame (NutraSweet), Saccharin, and Maltodextrin

#1 Omega 3's: Chia or flax seeds, safe fish (See list), Green vegetables, Omega supplement	Vegetable, Nut, and Seed oils, Commercial meat and dairy, Oils in packaged foods
Monounsaturated (Omega-9) fats: Extra virgin olive oil, avocados, almonds, almond flour, hazelnuts or macadamia nuts. **Good Fat = Lose Fat & Inflammation**	Trans-fats **Bad Fat = Get Fat & Inflamed**
Olive oil based dressings	Vegetable or canola based, high sugar and calorie dressings
Coconut milk, coconut oil	
Good saturated fats from properly raised sources: Grass-fed beef (hamburger or steak), Pasture-raised and organic chicken and eggs, organic, grass-fed cheese and butter (raw is best if possible)	Limit fats from commercial meats and commercial dairy products
The best oils for cooking Coconut oil, butter oil. Olive oil (low temperature or cold only)	**Bad for cooking or use at any time** Vegetable, nut, or seed oil
Dairy Organic, grass-fed dairy products, goats milk dairy products, organic, raw butter and cheese, grass-fed, un-denatured whey powder	Any non-organic commercial dairy product. No commercial cheese, milk, whey
Beverages: Purified water (can add lemon), lemon and Stevia, cucumber slices, sparkling water (with lemon or lime), fresh vegetable juices, smoothies (see recipes)	**No Soda: Diet or Regular** No commercial dairy Limit caffeine and alcohol Apple, orange, grape, grapefruit juice, etc.

Meat from whole sources like pasture-raised, 100% grass-fed and finished beef, and free-range chicken	Commercial feed and grain-eating animals injected with growth hormones, steroids, and antibiotics Worse: Processed meats Pork and pork products
Wild fish from the "safe fish" list	Farm-raised fish, shell fish, and other fish from the toxic list
Dairy and eggs from whole, naturally-fed sources	Dairy products and eggs from commercial, feed cows, and chickens
Seeds: raw flax, hemp, pumpkin, and sunflower seeds	Large amounts of seeds Large amounts of roasted seeds
Moderate amounts of raw walnuts, almonds, cashews	Large amounts! Avoid roasting nuts as well
Small amounts of fermented soy products	Processed and excessive soy products, i.e., soy milk, soy protein, tofu, etc.
Modest amounts of Legumes: including beans, peas, and lentils (see our soaking/sprouting instructions in the Appendix)	Large amounts are a problem due to anti-nutrients.
Good Protein for Vegans: • Moderate Legumes: beans and lentils • Raw nuts and seeds • Vegan plant protein supplement: rice, hemp, peas • Fermented soy product	**Do not Eat or Drink Soy!**

APPENDIX II

Carb Counter: A Chart of Lower-Glycemic Index Carbohydrate Sources

FOOD	SERVING SIZE	TOTAL CARBOHYDRATES	TOTAL FIBER
FRUIT			
Apples (with skin)	1 medium-sized apple	25	4
Asian Pears	1 whole medium fruit	13	4
Avocado (California)	1 whole, without skin	12	9
Bananas	Medium (7-8" long)	27	3
Blackberries	1 cup	15	8
Blueberries	1 cup	21	4
Dates (Deglet Nour)	1 cup chopped	110	12
Grapefruit	Full fruit (6-8" diameter)	26	4
Grapes	1 cup	16	1
Honeydew melon	1 cup balled	16	1
Kiwis	1 cup	26	5
Lemons	1 fruit	8	2
Limes	1 lime	7	2
Mangoes	1 cup sliced	28	3

Melon (Cantaloupe)	1 cup balled	16	2
Oranges (Florida)	1 large whole fruit	17	4
Peach	1 large whole	17	3
Pineapple	1 cup, chunked	22	2
Plums	1 fruit	8	1
Pomegranate	1 fruit	53	11
Red cherries	1 cup, without pits	19	2
Strawberries	1 cup whole strawberries	11	3
Tomato	1 large whole	7	2
Watermelon	1 cup balled	12	1
VEGETABLES			
Artichokes (boiled and prepared)	1 medium artichoke	14	10
Arugula	1 cup, uncooked leaves	1	0
Banana peppers	1 medium whole pepper	2	2
Broccoli	1 cup chopped	6	2
Brussels sprouts	1 cup	8	3
Cabbage	1 cup chopped	5	2

Carrots	1 cup chopped	12	4
Cucumber	1 cup chopped	3	1
Garlic	3 cloves	3	0
Green beans	1 cup	8	4
Green leaf lettuce	1 cup shredded	1	0
Green peas	1 cup	21	7
Jalapeno peppers	1 cup sliced	6	3
Kale	1 cup chopped	7	1
Onions	1 cup chopped	15	3
Potato	1 whole potato	27	2
Pumpkin	1 cup, cubed	8	1
Red peppers	1 medium whole pepper	7	2
Spinach	1 cup, uncooked leaves	1	1
Summer squash	1 cup sliced	4	1
Sweet corn	1 medium ear	26	3
Sweet potato (cooked, with skin)	1 medium whole	24	4
Swiss chard	1 cup	1	1

NUTS AND LEGUMES			
Almonds	1 cup whole	30	17
Black beans	1 cup	23	8
Brazil nuts	1 cup whole	16	10
Chickpeas (Garbanzo beans)	1 cup	54	11
Lima beans	1 cup	40	9
Macadamia nuts	1 cup whole	19	11
Peanuts	1 cup	24	12
LOW-GLYCEMIC, HIGH-FIBER GRAINS			
Brown rice (cooked)	1 cup	45	4
Multi-grain bread	2 slices	22	4
Oatmeal	1 cup	103	17
Quinoa (cooked)	1 cup	39	5
Rye bread	2 slices	30	4

APPENDIX III

Protein Counter

Animal Foods
Land

Beef average	7g per ounce
4 ounces hamburger	28g
6 ounces steak	42g
3 ounces leg of lamb	22g
3 ounces chicken breast, no skin	24g
4 ounces pork loin	29g
3 ounces cooked ground pork	22g
1 slice bacon	3g
1 slice Canadian bacon	5.5g

Sea

Fish average	6g per ounce
6 ounce can of Tuna	40g
4 ounces Mahi Mahi	20g
4 ounces Salmon	24-25g
4 ounces Tilapia	23g
3 ounces shrimp	11g
1 ounce Sardines	7g

Eggs and dairy

Large egg	6g
1 cup milk	8g
½ cup cottage cheese	15g
1 cup yogurt	8-12g (check label)

Soft cheeses (Mozzarella, Brie, etc.)	6g/ounce
Medium cheeses (Cheddar, Swiss)	7.5g/ounce
Hard cheeses (Parmesan)	10g/ounce

Beans, nuts, legumes, and seeds

2 tablespoons peanut butter	8g
¼ cup Almonds	8g
¼ cup Peanuts	9g
¼ cup Cashews	5g
¼ cup Sunflower seeds	6g
¼ cup Pumpkin seeds	8g
¼ cup Flax seeds	8g
½ cup cooked beans	7-10g average

You may remember from earlier chapters that your body generally can't properly metabolize a helping of protein that exceeds 20-30 grams in a meal. In order to get that amount, you can check out some of the following protein-rich foods and the serving sizes it will take to get that much protein:

How to get 20-30 grams of Protein in a meal

Eggs	4-5 eggs, depending on size
Beef	A 3-4 oz. hamburger patty or beef filet each offers 23-32 grams of protein
Untrimmed steak	3-4 ounces offers 21-28 grams of protein
Leg of lamb	3-4 ounces offers 22-30 grams
Chicken breast, no skin	3-4 ounces offers 24-32 grams
Turkey	3-4 ounces offers 22-30 grams
Mahi Mahi	4-6 ounces offers 20-30 grams
Tilapia	4-6 ounces offers 22.7-31 grams
Salmon	4-6 ounces offers 24-32 grams

Tuna	6 ounce can offers 40 grams of protein
Shrimp	6 ounces offers 22 grams of protein
Milk	Three cups offers 24 grams
Cottage cheese	½ cup offers 15 grams
Soft cheeses (Mozzarella, Brie)	6 grams per ounce
Medium Cheese (Cheddar, Swiss)	7-8 grams per ounce
Hard cheese (Parmesan)	10 grams per ounce

APPENDIX IV

Soaking and Sprouting Instructions
Making Nuts, Grains, Seeds, and Beans More Edible

Nuts, grains, beans, and seeds are designed to stay alive and intact until time to sprout and grow. As a result, nature has placed within them an internal defense system that causes these foods to be anti-nutrients or even toxic in high doses. These things have become a common part of our diets, but they contain substances that can inhibit food-digesting enzymes and block the absorption of key minerals.

If you think of proper growing conditions, these seed-based foods become wet over time, so they can germinate and reproduce themselves as the plant foods we eat. In a nutshell, pun-intended, this is why we need to soak and sprout these nutrients to make them safer to eat. As they go through the soaking and sprouting process, the substances that create problems in human health can be reduced or eliminated.

Soaking nuts, beans, seeds and sprouting grains also serves to increase the presences of vitamins (particularly B vitamins), reduce the presence of unhealthy tannins and phylates, enhance the production of digestive enzymes, break down unhealthy gluten, and provide several other benefits.

Below are the basics to soaking and sprouting. Other options can be easily found on-line. It's a popular topic. Given the challenges related to these foods, these should be eaten in moderation.

Some Basic Nut, Seed, and Bean Soaking Instructions

- Use water with approximately 1 tablespoon of salt. Some methods recommend adding an acidic agent like lemon juice. Beans can also be soaked in vinegar.
- Minimum time to see results is 7 hours with best results coming in 12 to 24 hours.
- Eat nuts and seeds wet or dried in a dehydrator.

Basic Sprouting Instructions

1. Rinse the grains

2. Place them in a glass or stainless steel container, and fill with warm water until the water is 2 to 3 inches above the grain.

3. Soak the grains for 12 hours/overnight.

4. After the time is up, pour out the water through a screen filter or a mesh cloth, and leave them moist in the container.

5. Rinse the grains multiple times, stirring so you get all of them evenly.

6. Rinse the grains occasionally over the course of 1-3 days until you see the buds appearing as they begin to sprout.

7. Drain them, refrigerate, or use a dehydrator if you're going to grind for use as flour.

Dream Center Run for Hope Foundation

PERSONALIZE YOUR CAUSE

Ensure your audience understands why the cause of human trafficking is important, rather than making it only about the marathon.

Here are some quick facts about human trafficking that will also help you:
- $90 is the average cost of a human slave
- There are 27 million people in slavery worldwide
- Odds of rescue are one in a hundred... 99% are never rescued
- 800,000 people are trafficked across international borders each year
- The average age of entry into prostitution is 12-14 years of age

DREAM BIG AND SET GOALS

Here are some tips to help in setting your fundraising and training goals:

Be resolute and make a firm decision in your mind that you will stick to your goals and won't forget about them until you've achieved them.

Write them down and place that piece of paper somewhere where you can see it everyday, think and pray about them, ask God for the strength to be motivated and put in effort.

Make an action plan, stating what activities you would need to do to achieve your goals.

Involve others to keep you accountable and to encourage you.

Persist, persist, persist - try out different methods, learn and improve, focus and be patient.

Celebrate your successes!

Acknowledgements

Special thanks to:

My co-founder Dr. Greg Loman and the hundreds of Maximized Living doctors around the world committed to reaching 34 million people. They make programs like the Genesis Challenge possible and successful.

Pastors Tommy and Matthew Barnett for allowing the Maximized Living Foundation to serve at The Dream Center.

Bob Ramsey and Dr. April Smith: it's because of them that we've been helping thousands in the clinic and through the salad bar we've built at The Dream Center.

My wife, Dr. Sheri Lerner, and my children, Skylar, Nicole, and Cael. They are the inspiration I have for taking care of myself and wanting to see millions of other dads and moms do the same.

About the Author

Dr. Ben Lerner is the founder of Maximized Living and is a *New York Times* bestselling author of over a dozen books and curriculum including *Body by God*, *Maximized Metabolix*, *The Cancer Killers*, and *One-Minute Wellness*, with Dr. Greg Loman.

Dr. Lerner's work at Maximized Living is to help people change the way they view and manage their health, offering doctors the tools to run practices that transform communities through the 5 Essentials.

The Mission of Maximized Living is to *avoid unnecessary human suffering by changing the practice of health care through the 5 Essentials*—Maximized Mind™; Maximized Nerve Supply™; Maximized Quality Nutrition™; Maximized Oxygen and Lean Muscle™; and Minimized Toxins™. Their Vision is simple: *through an unshakable commitment to living and sharing the 5 Essentials, 34 million people will enjoy the health needed to experience their potential.*

Early in his life, Dr. Lerner suffered from debilitating joint pain and developed a bleeding ulcer as a side effect of prescription anti-inflammatories. The fact that he could no longer take the medications led him to a chiropractor and nutritionist who changed his life.

In 1995, he was named the first official chiropractor for the USA Wrestling World Team, and he traveled with USAW to the Atlanta and Sidney Olympic Games, as well as eight world championships, eventually working as a doctor for professional teams like the Orlando Magic.

He now co-chairs the Sports Performance Council, which has provided performance care and education to many professional and world teams and athletes. He focuses a great deal of his time on the Maximized Living Foundation and its work to provide the underserved with the same quality and quantity of care provided in Maximized Living's for-profit clinics around the world.

Dr. Lerner lives in Florida with his wife, Dr. Sheri Lerner, and their three children, Skylar, Nicole, and Cael.